Amira El-Houfey
Mahmoud   Ammar

Nursing and infection control strategies

Amira El-Houfey
Mahmoud Ammar

Nursing and infection control strategies

LAP LAMBERT Academic Publishing

Impressum / Imprint

Bibliografische Information der Deutschen Nationalbibliothek: Die Deutsche Nationalbibliothek verzeichnet diese Publikation in der Deutschen Nationalbibliografie; detaillierte bibliografische Daten sind im Internet über http://dnb.d-nb.de abrufbar.
Alle in diesem Buch genannten Marken und Produktnamen unterliegen warenzeichen-, marken- oder patentrechtlichem Schutz bzw. sind Warenzeichen oder eingetragene Warenzeichen der jeweiligen Inhaber. Die Wiedergabe von Marken, Produktnamen, Gebrauchsnamen, Handelsnamen, Warenbezeichnungen u.s.w. in diesem Werk berechtigt auch ohne besondere Kennzeichnung nicht zu der Annahme, dass solche Namen im Sinne der Warenzeichen- und Markenschutzgesetzgebung als frei zu betrachten wären und daher von jedermann benutzt werden dürften.

Bibliographic information published by the Deutsche Nationalbibliothek: The Deutsche Nationalbibliothek lists this publication in the Deutsche Nationalbibliografie; detailed bibliographic data are available in the Internet at http://dnb.d-nb.de.
Any brand names and product names mentioned in this book are subject to trademark, brand or patent protection and are trademarks or registered trademarks of their respective holders. The use of brand names, product names, common names, trade names, product descriptions etc. even without a particular marking in this work is in no way to be construed to mean that such names may be regarded as unrestricted in respect of trademark and brand protection legislation and could thus be used by anyone.

Coverbild / Cover image: www.ingimage.com

Verlag / Publisher:
LAP LAMBERT Academic Publishing
ist ein Imprint der / is a trademark of
OmniScriptum GmbH & Co. KG
Heinrich-Böcking-Str. 6-8, 66121 Saarbrücken, Deutschland / Germany
Email: info@lap-publishing.com

Herstellung: siehe letzte Seite /
Printed at: see last page
ISBN: 978-3-659-66634-6

Zugl. / Approved by: Post-doctoral, Assiut University, Egypt. 2014

Author's Affiliations

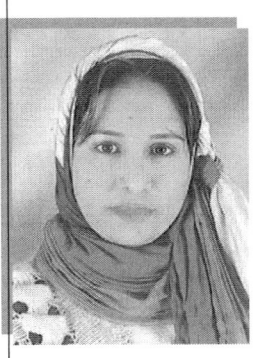

Dr . Amira Abdallah El- Houfey

- Lecturer of Community Health Nursing, Faculty of Nursing , Assiut University, Egypt.

- PhD. in Community Health Nursing, excellent degree (2012), Faculty of Nursing, Assiut University, Assiut City. Egypt.

- Master Degree in Community Health Nursing, excellent degree (2008), Faculty of Nursing, Assiut University, Assiut City. Egypt.

  - Baccalaureate of Nursing, excellent degree (2001), Faculty of Nursing, Assiut University, Assiut City. Egypt
- Mobile: (+)201063113342.
- Email: amiraelhoufey@yahoo.com
- Place of birth: Kafer El-Sheik City, Dissouk District, Egypt.
- Date of birth: 1- 10- 1980.

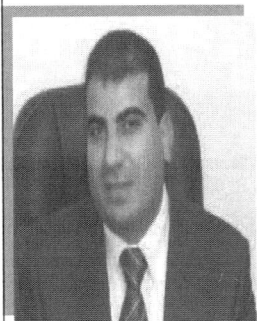

Dr . Mahmoud Mohamed Ammar

- Lecturer of Prosthodontics and Dental Implantology at Faculty of Dental Medicine, Al Azhar University (Assuit Branch), Egypt.

- -Ph.D in Removable Prosthodontics, Faculty of Dental Medicine, Al Azhar University (2008), Cairo, Egypt.

- Master's Degree in Removable Prosthodontics, Faculty of Dental Medicine, Al Azhar University (2003), Cairo , Egypt.

- B.D.S. in Dental Medicine, Faculty of Dental Medicine, Al Azhar University (1996),Cairo, Egypt.

- Email: dr_3mmar3@yahoo.com

- Place of birth: Al kusssia District, Assuit , Egypt.
- Date of birth :23-11-1972.

Contents

List of abbreviation:

Abbreviation	Meaning
AIDS	Acquired immunodeficiency syndrome.
BSI	Body Substance Isolation.
CDC	Center for disease control and prevention.
DHCP	Dental health-care personnel.
DHCWs	Dental Health Care Workers.
HICPAC	Hospital Infection Control Practices Advisory Committee
HBV	Hepatitis B virus.
HCP	Health-Care Personnel.
HCWs	Health Care Workers.
HCV	Hepatitis C virus.
HIV	Human immunodeficiency virus.
IC	Infection control.
ICN	Infection control nurse.
MOHP	Ministry of Health and Population
NAP	National AIDS Program.
OSHA	Occupational Safety and Health Administration.
TB	Tuberculosis.
UNAIDS	United Nations Programme on HIV/AIDS.
UP	Universal Precautions.
WHO	World Health Organization.

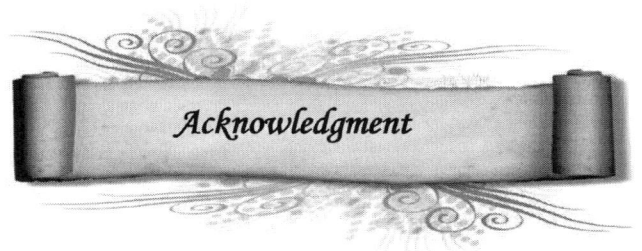

Acknowledgment

First and foremost, I feel always indebted to (ALLAH) the kindest and most merciful for all countless gifts have offered us

Pursuing this work has not been easy for him, so we wish to express our sincere appreciation to all members who love and encouraged us much, many thanks to Dr. Neama El Magrabi, Dr. Shokria Labeeb and for Dr. Kawther Fadel who helped us in revising this work. These words are not enough to convey our deep heart feelings:

To our parent'
To husband/ wife

To our daughters/ suns

To all members of our family and close friends

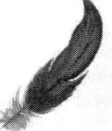

Dr .Amira A. El- Houfey & Dr .Mahmoud M. Ammar

2014

Introduction:

The world is facing an outbreak of the highly contagious infectious diseases; and the dental health care providers have the responsibility of protecting their patients from contracting these infections from dental treatment. They themselves should also be highly vigilant towards contracting the same diseases from their patients *(Wong, 2003)*.

Infection control forms an important part of practice for all health care professions and remains one of the most cost-beneficial medical interventions available *(McCarthy et al, 1999)*. However, there are still uncertainties in aspects of cross-infection and infection control in dentistry *(Pistorius et al, 2002)*. Infection control practices in developing countries have not been widely documented *(Morries et al, 1996)*.

Infection means invasion and multiplication of pathogenic microorganisms in tissues or on surfaces of the body where they can harm the host and cause adverse effects *(Green and Ottoson, 1994, Ayliffe et al, 1992, and Ajemian and Castle, 1987)*. Infection may be localized or systematic, localized infection is most common in areas of skin or mucous membrane breakdown such as wounds, and mouth lesions *(Potter and Perry, 1998)*. On the other hand systematic infection usually develop after failing of treatment for localized infection and it causes generalized symptoms such as fever, fatigue, malaise, nausea, vomiting, and enlarged lymphnodes *(Andreoll et al, 1998)*.

Cross-infection is defined as the transmission of infectious agents between patients and staff within a clinical environment *(Samarnayake et al, 2002)*. Dental patients and Dental Health Care Workers (DHCWs) may be exposed to a variety of microorganisms via blood, oral, or respiratory secretions *(Malik, 2002)*.

In recent years, the danger of transmitting infection to the dental team or other patients has become apparent, particularly with the threat of acquired immunodeficiency syndrome (AIDS) and hepatitis. Universal precautions (UP), including protective attire and barrier technique are strongly recommended and often required by law *(Newman et al, 2003)*.

Dental health-care personnel (DHCP) refers to all paid and unpaid personnel in the dental health-care setting who might be occupationally exposed to infectious materials, including body substances and contaminated supplies, equipment, environmental surfaces, water, or air. (DHCP) includes dentists, dental hygienists, dental assistants, students and trainees, contractual personnel, housekeepers, and maintenance personnel *(Kohn et al, 2004)*.

The hospital is an ideal environment for transmission of infection as many numbers of patients with similar diseases and susceptibilities share contact with many health care workers. The patients or client may acquire the infection during or after hospitalization *(Bennett and Brachman, 1998)*, i.e. this infection is neither present nor incubating at the time of admission *(Salamaa, 1996)*. This type of infection is called nosocomial or hospital acquired infection, and it affect not only patients and health care workers but also any one who gets in contact with a hospital, including visitors, sales person and delivery personnel *(Bennett and Brachman, 1998)*.

Nosocomial infections constitute a major public health problem because of increase morbidity and mortality among hospitalized patients. In 1996 hospital acquired infection occurred at rate of 5-10 per 100 admission in United States *(Bannister et al, 2000 and Courtenary, 1997)*.

There are four major categories of nosocomial infections these include surgical wound infections, urinary tract infections, respiratory infections, and blood steam infections *(Abdullah, 1996)*.

Nowadays, there is an increase in the prevalence rate of blood borne infections. Blood borne pathogens can be transmitted through, blood, wound secretion, cerebrospinal fluids, peritoneal fluids, and amniotic fluids. More over there is an increase in the number of individual presenting for care of symptomatically infected with blood borne pathogens such as Human Immunodeficiency Virus (HIV), Hepatitis B virus (HBV), Hepatitis C virus (HCV) and Delta Hepatitis *(Abdel All, 1998)*.

Hepatitis C virus has already become a major public health problem. The incidence of HCV is not well known. But the prevalence studies estimated by World Health Organization (WHO) showed that 3% of world populations are infected with HCV *(World Health Reports, 1998)*. In the United States 3.5 million people 1.8% have antibody to hepatitis *(Ryan and Ray, 2004)*.

In Egypt, about 3 million people are treated yearly in Ministry of Health dental clinics *(Ministry of Health and Population, Egypt Infection control Program, Infection Control Office, WHO Regional Office for the Eastern Mediterranean and internet publisher)*.

Studies in the Middle East showed that the prevalence of HBVs ranged from 4% to 5% in Iraq, 2.6% to 10% in Jordan *(Toukan, 1997 and WHO Regional Office, 1995)*, and 19.6 % in Egypt *(El-Sayed et al, 1997)*.

As a result of studies have been performed, investigating HCV risks in dental professionals, among dentists of New York City it was found that 1.75 percent are infected *(Molinari,1999)*.

HIV infection is wide spread, an estimated 36.1 million adults and children have AIDS worldwide *(WHO, 2001)*. In the United States recent years incidence rate have stabilized at about 40,000 cases per year *(US Department of Health and Human Services, 2000)*. In 2004, the Joint United Nations Programme on HIV/AIDS (UNAIDS) estimated that 12,000 adults and children were living with HIV/AIDS in Egypt. The National AIDS Program (NAP) stated that by the end of 2004 a total of 2,115 cases of HIV/AIDS had been reported to the Ministry of Health and Population. There are differences between reported cases and estimates that indicate weaknesses in the surveillance system and barriers to HIV *(UNAIDS, 2005)*.

Infection control (IC) strategies must be followed routinely for all patients. The universal precaution for dental team entail the employment of various personal protective barrier techniques such as gloves, gown, face mask, and protective eye wear, avoiding injury from sharp instruments, hand washing, disinfection of dental unit surface and proper disposal of wastes *(Mailk,2002)*.

Every person goes to dental clinics, healthy and unhealthy male or female, child and adult. Although identification of risks to dental health care workers has been explored in several industrialized nations, very little data is available from developing countries *(Fasunloro and Owotade, 2004)*.

In Egypt, HCV infection rate is 25%. Egypt has a higher incidence of HCV infection than any other country in the world *(Arthur et al, 1997)*. Several studies suggest that exposure to dental procedures is a risk factor for HCV in Egypt *(Ministry of Health and population, Egypt Infection control Program, infection control office, and WHO Regional Office for the Eastern Mediterranean)*. Several studies have documented blood borne pathogen transmission in the health care facilities in Egypt. Between 1994 and 2000 it was related to poor adherence to standard infection control precautions *(Talaat et al, 2003)*.

DHCWs had already recognized the potential of transmission of diseases in every directions from dental team to patients and from patients to dental team. Hepatitis B virus (HBV) had been well documented from dentists to patients, as well as herpes transmission from dental hygienists to patients *(Gluck and Morganstein, 2003)*.

The majority of (DHCP) infected with a blood borne virus have the opportunity for transmission of infection is greatest from patient to DHCP, who frequently encounter patient blood and blood-contaminated saliva during dental procedures *(Centers for Disease Control and Prevention, 2003)*.

Many countries in the Eastern Mediterranean Region still had a lack of effective infection control programs *(Talaat et al, 2003)*. International researches reported that health care workers had a 20 to 40 time's greater risk of contracting hepatitis C virus than HIV from an accidental needle stick *(Frotline, 2000)*.

Health care workers represent approximately 2% to 6% of reported cases from hepatitis B virus in the United States; that are a major infectious occupational hazards to health care workers *(Kane et al, 1989 in Gluck and Morganstein, 2003)*.

Transmission of tuberculosis in dental practices is most likely from patients without recognized diseases not receiving anti -TB (tuberculosis) therapy, inadequate ventilation and contact with patients, in small, enclosed area as well that can play a part in transmission of TB disease *(Gluck and Morganstein, 2003)*.

Community health nurses have an important role in the prevention and control of communicable diseases, the primary prevention methods of mass media, one-on-one education, and encouraging immunization compliance for all people. Secondary prevention includes case finding and screening tests. Tertiary prevention is needed to ensure additional people are not infected; this is accomplished through isolation, and encourages universal precaution practices among health care workers and the safe handling and control of infectious wastes *(Allender and Spradley, 2001)*. Nurses and clients must be educated on the types of infection and modes of transmission. IC is vital to health care delivery systems and to communities *(Daniels, 2004)*.

Infections acquired in health care settings have emerged as an important public health problem and are a leading cause of morbidity and mortality worldwide; they affect both developed and poor resource countries and constitute a significant burden both for the patient and for the health care system *(World Health Organization Report, 2002)*.

IC has become a major concern of patient regulatory agencies, and health care workers in the practices of dentistry; the dental team should have been practicing infection control at all times *(Frommer and Stabulas - Savage, 2005)*.

1) An overview of Infection Control (IC):

Historically, three forms of body fluid precautions have been practiced in Canada. Before 1987, facilities used blood labeling precautions *(Health and Welfare Canada, 1985)*; then universal precaution *(Health Canada, 1987)*; and Body Substance Isolation (BSI) *(Lynch et al, 1987)*. In 1997, new integrated blood borne pathogen protocols were developed and introduced with the publication of Preventing the Transmission of Blood borne Pathogens in Health Care and Public Service Settings *(Health Canada, 1997)*. The term standard infection control precautions and protection against (HCV) has been included under this infection control umbrella *(Occupational Safety and Health Administration, 2001)*.

The procedures of (IC) followed today in dentistry are radically different from those followed before 1986 when CDC published its original infection-control guidelines *(Centers for Disease Control, 1986)*. Many infection-control procedures followed in dentists' offices are scientifically based and required by law and legal organization *(Shulman and Brehm, 2001)*.

Center for Disease Control and Prevention (CDC):

The early guidelines did not specifically address dental care but outlined suggested precautions to be used when dealing with patients with AIDS, such as the use of gloves, refraining from bending or recapping needles, the use of gown, and the use of extraordinary care to prevent injury, the recommended use of procedures already known to be appropriate for persons infected with (HBV). The first actual recommendation for (DHCW) in 1983 stated the following: Personnel should wear gloves, masks, and protective eyewear when performing dental or oral surgical procedure and instruments used in the mouth of patients should be sterilized *(Acquired Immunodeficiency Syndrome "AIDS", 1983)*.

State of the art of (IC) guidelines for dentistry did not merge until April 18, 1986, when CDC published " Recommended infection control practices for dentistry ".These recommendations were based on the used of a common set of infection control strategies to be used routinely in the care of all patients in dental practices. It was emphasized that diseases transmission in either direction, patient to DHCW or DHCW to patients *(Recommended Infection Control Practices for Dentistry, 1986)*.

Other major guidelines for infection control were released in 1987 and 1988 from the CDC and referred, in part especially to DHCW *(Recommendations for prevention of HIV transmission in health-care settings,1987; and Update: UP for prevention transmission of HIV, HBV, and other blood borne pathogens in health care settings , 1988)*.

The guidelines for dentistry, updated and released in July 1993, represent a logical progression of knowledge in (IC) and exposure management and provide a clear understanding of diseases transmission mechanisms and the associated risks. In addition, there is a shift from the earlier emphasis on blood borne disease transmission to include airborne diseases now, such as Mycobacterium tuberculosis and other respiratory illnesses *(Recommended Infection Control Practices for Dentistry, 1993)*.

The relevance of (UP) to other aspects of disease transmission was recognized, and in 1996 CDC expanded the concept and changed the term to standard precautions. Standard precautions integrate and expand the elements of (UP) into a standard of care designed to protect HCP and patients from pathogens that can be spread by blood or any other body fluid, excretion, or secretion *(Garner and Hospital Infection Control Practices Advisory Committee "HICPAC", 1996)*. Standard precautions apply to contact with blood, all body fluids, secretions, and excretions except sweat, regardless of whether they contain visible blood, nonintact skin; and mucous membranes *(CDC Guideline for Isolation, 2004)*. Saliva has always been considered a potentially infectious material in dental infection control; thus no operational difference exists in clinical dental practice between universal precautions and standard precautions *(Centers for Disease Control and Prevention, 2003)*.

2) Infection control goal and rational:

The goal of (IC) is to create and maintain safe clinical environment for eliminating the potential for disease transmission from clinician to client, client to clinician, and from client to client *(Darby and Walsh, 2003)*. Infection control and prevention are models for quality management and patient safety *(Pittet, 2005)*.

Elimination or reduction of the spread from all types of microorganisms is the duty of every dental practitioner to care of all patients, including those with infectious diseases *(Mailk, 2002)*. The dental team also has ethical and legal professional responsibility for implementing infection control measures for elimination of the spread of infection *(Samarnayake et al, 2002)*.

Members of the dental team (dentists and their assistants) are working in close contact with their patients. Either they themselves or the patients can transmit the infection to each other since the potential carriers in the community are not identifiable. The patients in as much as members of the dental team themselves can be potential carriers. Therefore, we should treat one another as potential infection carriers and take universal precautionary measures *(Wong, 2003)*.

DHCWs are at potential risk of exposure and possible infection from a variety of microbial diseases, so that it is essential to protect themselves and their patients *(Wilson and Kornman, 2003)*. Specific failings in recommended infection control procedures vary from country to country *(Gordon et al, 2001)*.

The main objective is to protect patients and (DHCP) against the risks of cross infection in the dental surgery environment. The major risk of infection to dental health care personnel is the repeated exposure to blood and to mixtures of blood and saliva, which may be contaminated with a wide variety of microorganisms including blood-borne viruses. Patients carrying blood-borne viruses may be asymptomatic and unaware of their carrier or infectious status. Medical histories and physical examinations cannot reliably identify all carriers of blood-borne diseases *(NZDA, 2002)*.

Moreover, *(Miller and Palenik, 1998)* stated that the goal of infection control is to eliminate or reduce the dose of microorganisms that may be shard between individuals or between individuals and contaminated surfaces.

Practices of (IC) aimed at reducing occupational risk include: routine use of aseptic techniques, immunization of care providers with available vaccine, use of protective barriers, use of appropriate engineering controls and other safety   measures, and use of effective sterilization and disinfection procedures *(Wilson and Kornman, 2003)*.

Qudeimat et al., (2006) stated that information regarding compliance with universal infection control precautions in the dental settings in the Middle East is scant.

Although the number of published studies concerning dental infection control have increased in recent years, questions regarding infection-control practices and their effectiveness remain unanswered so that more researches are needed in the field of infection control in dentistry *(Centers for Disease Control and Prevention, 2003)*.

3) Cross - infection:

The issue of cross-infection becomes an integral part of dental practice and a major concern to dentists and patients due to the increased risk of hepatitis and AIDS *(Morris et al, 1996)*. Dental care professionals routinely are at risk of cross-infection while providing care to patients *(Molinari, 2003)*.

Infection means an invasion and multiplication of microorganisms in body tissue that result in cellular injury. These microorganisms are called infectious agents; in addition communicable agents can be transmitted to clients by direct or indirect contact through vehicle or by air borne route and result in communicable disease *(While and Duncan, 2002)*.

Cross-infection is defined as the transmission of infectious agents between patients and staff within a clinical environment *(Malik, 2002)*. Transmission may result from person -to- person contact or via contaminated objects *(Samarnayake et al, 2002)*. Cross-contamination may be via direct or indirect means *(Darby and Walsh, 2003)*. Contaminated hands are a prime cause of cross- infection *(Potter and Perry, 2001)*.

Cross contamination is a severe problem that involves health professionals, especially in dentistry. The transmission of diseases during treatment between patients and dentists, auxiliary personnel and dental laboratory technicians can occur if preventive measures are not taken. The risk of cross-contamination in dental clinics as well as transmission of microorganisms have been reported in various studies *(Agostinho et al, 2004)*.

The use of effective infection control procedures and universal precaution in the dental office will prevent cross-contamination that could extend to dental office staff and patients *(American Dental Association, 1996)*.

There is no doubt that infections have been transmitted in the dental surgery from patient to dental staff, and from dental staff to patient. Mostly these have been blood- borne virus, airborne transmission, and other infections; so that organizations such as National Dental Association have produced guidelines for cross- infection control *(Scully and Cawson, 1998)*.

The provision of dental care is not without risk; of concern to both dental care workers and patients is the risk of exposure to blood borne pathogens, including hepatitis B and C viruses and human immunodeficiency virus injuries *(McCarthy and Britton, 2000)*. Since hepatitis C is a blood-borne infection and is transmitted efficiently by transfusion and by needle sharing, it stands to reason that an occupational risk for transmission of HCV in the health care setting might exist, including transmission from infected patients to staff, from patient to patient, and from infected providers to patients *(Henderson, 2003)*. Cross-infection (exogenous infection) with some of these organisms may occur from patients or members of staff either by contact or airborne *(Ayliffe et al, 2000)*.

The incidence of oral pathogens is higher on dental operatory environmental surfaces, compared with similar surfaces in non dental settings *(Hackeny et al, 1998)*.

Despite dental medicine has come along way in achieving the current level of (IC) success; many dental professional may not be aware of all the protective aspects of routinely applied precautions *(Wilson and Kornman, 2003)*. Many practical procedures carried out by nurses can be a source of infection; the nurse has both a legal and a professional duty of care toward patients, and must ensure that procedures are performed safely *(Huband et al, 2000)*.

A series of actions could considerably reduce the risk of cross-infection in dentistry such as, anti-sepsis, lying of barriers, use of conservatives, **d**isinfections, **d**isposal and **s**terilization (ABCDDS). This should be considered as important as hospital cross-contamination. There is no doubt that exposure of the dental staff and patients to high levels of microbial contamination leads to a high risk of infection *(Meiller et al, 2000)*. For effective (IC), every possible source of contamination should be submitted to ABCDDS actions before, during and after dental intervention *(June, 2003)*. The most effective method of preventing cross contamination is the use of personal barriers such as gloves, gown, protective clothing, eye glasses and environmental barriers such as decontaminate environmental surfaces, and sterilization of instruments *(Hackeny et al, 1998)*.

4) Infection chain:

(Potter and Perry, 2001) mentioned that the presence of a pathogen does not mean that an infection will begin. Development of an infection occurs in a cycle that depends on the presence of six following elements, an infection develops if this chain remain intact: an infectious agents or a pathogen.

- A reservoir or source of pathogen growth.

- A portal of exit from the reservoir.

- A mode of transmission.

- A portal of entry to host.

- A susceptible host.

- *Infectious agent:* The first link in the chain of infection is the microbial agent, which may be a bacterium, virus, fungus, or parasite. The ability of the infectious agents to cause disease depends on their pathogenicity, virulence, invasiveness, and specificity. Pathogenicity is the organism's ability to harm and cause diseases, virulence relates to the vigor by which the organisms can grow and multiply. Invasiveness describes the organism's ability to enter the tissues. Specificity refers to the organism's attraction to a specific host which may include humans *(Craven and Hirnle, 2007)*.

- *Reservoir:* Is the term used for any person, plant, animal, substance or location that provides nourishment for microorganism. Infection may be prevented by eliminating the causative organisms from the reservoir *(Smeltzer and Bare, 2004)*. A reservoir is a place where a pathogen survives but may or may not multiply *(Potter and Perry, 2001)*.

- *Portal of exit:* After microorganisms find a site to grow and multiply, they must find a portal of exit if they are to enter another host and cause diseases. Microorganisms can exit thought a variety of sites, such as the skin and mucous membrane, respiratory tract and blood *(Potter and Perry, 2001)*.

- *Mode of transmission:* The most frequent mode of transmission is contact transmission, airborne transmission and vehicle transmission which occur when an agent is transferred to susceptible host by animate object such as water, blood and drugs *(Daniels ,2004)*.

- *Portal of entry:* Portal of entry is the pathway the organism uses to gain entry to a susceptible host, these pathways are generally the same pathways used to exit a host, for example, skin and mucous membrane, percutaneously via blood, and respiratory tract *(Leahy and Kizilay, 1998)*.

- Susceptible host: When the person has a reduced immune response, this increases his susceptibility. The immune response describes a process which involves the body's natural defense against infection *(Centers for Disease Control and Prevention, 2003)*. A person's resistance to an infectious agent is enhanced by vaccine *(Potter and Perry, 2001)*.

5) Breaking the chain of infection

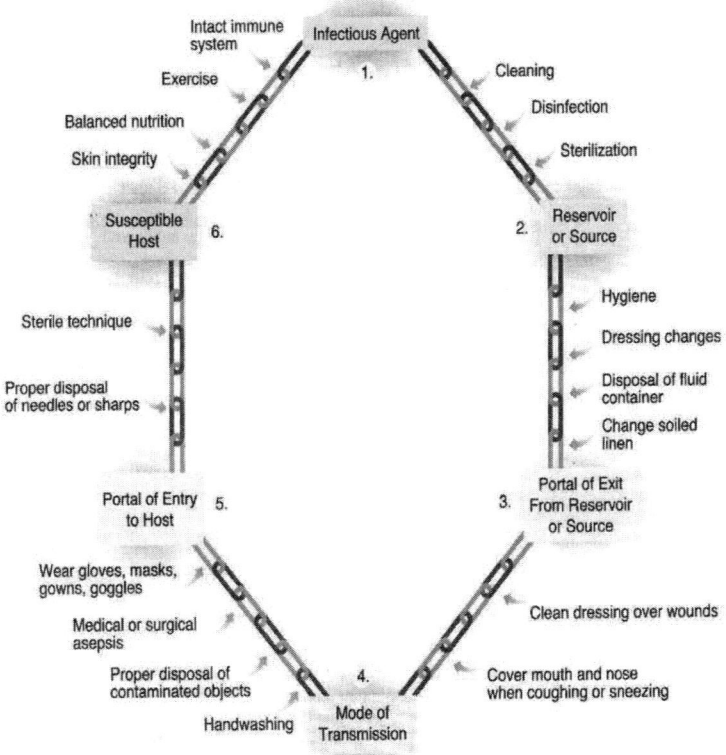

Figure (1): **Breaking the chain of infection; preventive measures follow each critical link in the chain of infection.** *(Cited from Daniels, 2004).*

6) Processing of instrument, gloves and other items :

Blood born pathogens such as HIV, HBV can be transmitted from one person (client or patient) to another through improperly processed needles, syringes and other invasive instruments, there fore, processing of instruments, gloves and other items is the basic infection prevention process which is essential to prevent infection. Processing instruments include: decontamination, cleaning and sterilization or high level disinfection *(World health organization, 1989)*.

Decontamination:- Is a process through which microorganisms such as HIV, HBV and HCV are removed or killed from instruments, equipments and other surface so that they become save to be handled and free from infection *(Greenand Ottoson, 1994)*.

Decontamination is a simple, inexpensive process which helps to protect both the staff members and clients or, patients from infection with blood borne pathogens. In order to increase protection, the person who deals with instruments during cleaning must wear a utility glove *(Speller et al, 1990)*.

The most recent direction from department of health and social security (DHSS) indicate that HIV, HBV and other blood born diseases such as HCV and Delta hepatitis new extremely sensitive to the action of hypochlorite. Thus they recommend the use of hypochlorite disinfection (chlorine- releasing disinfections), *(Bloomfield et al, 1990)*.

1) Decontamination of instruments:

Instruments are decontaminated by soaking in 0.5% chlorine solution for 10 minutes *(Shancon, 1998)*.

Preparation of 0.5% chlorine solutions differs from one country to another. Chlorine varies from 3.5% - 5%, in Egypt chlorine is available at 5% concentration. In order to prepare 0.5% chlorine solution from chlorine 5% one part of bleach added to mine parts of water *(Tietjem et al, 1992)*.

2- Decontamination of surfaces:

Large surfaces such as examination or operation which may come into contact with blood or body fluids should be decontaminations by wipping with a suitable disinfectant solution such as 0.5% chlorine solution before reuse or at least daily *(Tietjem et al, 1992)*.

3- Decontamination of blood spills:

Decontamination of blood spills can be achieved as the following, firstly wear utility gloves and absorb the blood spill with absorbent material (paper towel) and dispose it in container labeled with biohazard sign, then clean the area with 0.5% chlorine solution *(Joclaif, 1996)*.

7) Pathway of cross - contamination:

(Miller and Palenik, 1998) mentioned that a total office infection control program is designed to prevent or at least reduce the spread of disease agents from:

- Patient to dental team,

- Dental team to patient,

- Patient to patient,

- Dental office to community, including the dental team's family,

- And from community to patient.

8) Some 20Th Century accomplishments in Cross Infection Control:

(Molinari, 1999) mentioned that the 20Th century accomp-lishments in infection control are:

- Recognition of the relationship between microbial pathogens and the risk of occupational transmission of infectious diseases: blood borne, airborne, wound, acute, chronic.

- Developments and reinforcements of efficient aseptic techniques: hand washing procedures, class of antiseptics, infection control, cleaning procedures.

- Adaptation to the use of personal protective barriers during patient care : gloves, face mask, eye wear, clinic coat and gowns.

- Conversion from chemical immersion to heat sterilization procedures for instrument reprocessing.

- Application of universal precaution against blood borne disease as infection control standard for patient treatment.

- Adaptation of safer procedure to minimizing accidental exposure to contaminated sharp items.

- Developments and uses of newer technologies to prevent microbial contamination and facilitate better infection control: sterilizers, personal and equipment barriers, automated instruments cleaning equipment; reusable, heat stable dental instrumentation, single use of disposable needles.

- Discovery and development of antimicrobial antibiotics to treat clinical infections.

9) Source of infection in dentistry:

In dentistry the source of infection constitutes the following:

People with overt infections who liberate large numbers of organisms into their environment, e.g. droplets and discharges from the mouth or other portals as wounds, ulcer and sores in the skin; usually in routine clinical dentistry few patients are seem with acute disease *(Samarnayake et al, 2002)*.

Also people in the prodromal stage of certain infections, during this period the organisms multiplying without evidence of infection; the patient is highly infectious; viral infections such as measles, mumps and chicken pox, easily spread in this manner *(Malik, 2002)*.

People who are healthy carriers of pathogens that can be classified into:-

Asymptomatic carrier, gives no past history of infection; but individual may carry infective microbes in saliva, blood and other blood secretion ***(Malik, 2002)***; persons are colonized with an infectious agents but do not have the disease ***(Huband et al ,2000)***.

Convalescent carrier, in this stage the patient suffers from an acute illness and apparently recovers. This individual can be identified from the past history of infection ***(Malik, 2002);*** although blood and secretions of individual act as persistent reservoir of infective organization e.g. diphtheria or streptococcal sore throat. Clinician may be faced with either convalescent or a symptomatic carrier of (HBV) ***(Samarnayake et al, 2002)***.

10) Transmissible diseases:

The oral cavity harbors microorganisms with potential to transmit a wide spectrum of infectious agents. Dental professionals are therefore at risk for any orally transmissible diseases from the blood or saliva of the patients they treat them. In addition, the trauma of some dental procedures and mixing of blood and saliva enhance the risk of blood borne diseases transmission ***(Gluck and Morganstein, 2003)***.

Blood borne viruses accounts for most cases of occupational infection described in the literature because of their prevalence among patients and the severity of the infections they cause *(Tarantola et al, 2006)*.

HCWs engaged in direct patient care are at considerable risk of acquiring hepatitis B, C and HIV at their place of work through exposure to contaminated blood and body fluids while executing their routine of patient care *(Gustavo et al, 2006)*.

The increase profile of infections arising from blood-borne viruses such as (HIV), (HBV) and (HCV) since the mid-1980s has resulted in detailed scrutiny of infection control procedures within dentistry. A wide range of organisms poses a threat in the dental setting. However, of the blood-borne viruses, (HBV) is by far the most infectious and it is fortunate that a vaccine exists to protect dental staff. However most patients are not similarly protected and there also exists the potential for transmission of HCV and HIV to both patients and staff members *(Gordon et al, 2001)*.

Since the mid-1980s, recommended measures such as the wearing of gloves, masks, and the autoclaving of handpieces have been reviewed regularly with additional recommendations continually being issued in the light of new scientific evidence. In particular, the concept of universal infection control has become accepted as the best practice, whereby all patients are treated as potential carriers of pathogenic micro-organisms *(Gordon et al, 2001)*.

Dental patients and (DHCP) can be exposed to pathogenic microorganisms including cytomegalovirus (CMV), HBV, HCV, herpes simplex virus types 1 and 2, HIV, Mycobacterium tuberculosis, staphylococci, streptococci, and other viruses and bacteria that colonize or infect the oral cavity and respiratory tract system *(Centers for Disease Control and Prevention, 2003)*. The transmissible diseases currently of the greatest concern to the dental professional are HBV, HIV, HCV and Mycobacterium tuberculosis *(Gluck and Morganstein, 2003)*.

11) Mode of transmission of dental diseases:

The organisms can be transmitted in dental settings through: direct contact of tissues with blood, oral fluids. This is the least common mode, e.g. an ungloved practitioner with a cut on the finger performing an extraction (Samarnayake et al, 2002).

Indirect contact with contaminated objects; indirect cross-contamination occurs when instruments, equipments or environmental surfaces are contaminated with a client's oral fluids, either through touch or spatter. Contamination occurs when a container of dental material is handled with contamination gloves which is not disinfected, and then handled again with gloved hands when treating another client or from charts handled with a contaminated gloved hand *(Darby and Walsh, 2003)*. Contact of conjunctival, nasal, or oral mucosa with droplets (e.g., spatter) containing microorganisms generated from an infected person and propelled a short distance (e.g., by coughing, sneezing, or talking); and inhalation of airborne microorganisms that can remain suspended in the air for long periods *(Centers for Disease Control and Prevention, 2003)*.

Percutaneous exposure to blood, blood products, and infectious body fluids present the greatest risk for transmission of infection in the health care setting *(Kandeel et al, 2003)*. Direct inoculation into cuts and abrasions of unprotected skin or mucosa via contaminated sharps or instruments are other factors *(Malik, 2002)*.

Percutaneous injuries among (DHCP) usually occur outside the patient's mouth, that caused by burs, syringe needles, laboratory knives, and other sharp instruments *(Younai et al, 2001)*.

Transmission of infection within dental surgery may occur by direct contact of tissues with secretions or blood, from droplets containing infectious agents, or via contaminated sharps or dental instruments that have been improperly sterilized *(Mousa et al, 1997)*.

12) Infection Control Procedures in Dental Health-Care Settings:

A) Medical history:

The collection of an accurate medical history is part of good clinical practices and helpful is in the identification of immunocompromised patients. However, medical history can provide useful information of previous infectious diseases, the clinician must be aware that it *"does not"* allow for the categorization of patient into "high risk "and "low risk " *(Wray et al, 2003)*.

A thorough medical history should be obtained for all patients at the first visit and updated regularly. Medical history questionnaires alongside direct questioning and discussion between the dentist and the patient are recommended. Discussions should be conducted in an environment that permits the disclosure of sensitive personal information. The medical history information should be retained as part of the patient's dental records. The medical history and examination may not identify asymptomatic carriers of infectious disease and universal precautions must be adopted. This means that the same infection control procedures must be used for all patients *(British Dental Association Advisory Service, 2003)*.

All staff is trained in the proper management of records, including keeping them away from the public view in the front office, safe storage, and maintenance due to appropriate data protection legislation *(Samarnayake et al, 2002)*.

B) Immunization:

Vaccination is the administration of a vaccine or toxoid, which confers active immunity by stimulating the body to produce antibodies *(Nies and Ewen, 2001)*.

Vaccination (immunization) is an important tool in preventing the transmission of diseases, maintaining immunity to vaccine -preventable diseases is an important part of any (IC) program *(Silverman et al, 2001)*.

Health care providers are at increased risk to exposure to viral hepatitis B, and C so that vaccination for population who are at risk of hepatitis B is recommends *(Ewen, 2002)*. Most exposures to infectious agents in the dental setup are accidental and can be avoided by using safe work practices and following infection control guidelines. However, because some exposures are not preventable, immunization and appropriate post exposure management become the key defense *(McCarthy and Britton, 2000)*.

Hospital personnel are at risk for contracting and transmitting vaccine- preventable diseases maintenance of current immunization status is a good health practices *(Craven and Hirnle, 2007)*.

The optimal use of vaccine can prevent transmission of diseases and can help eliminate unnecessary work restrictions. Vaccination prevents illness and is far less cost and effective than individual case management or out break control. It is known that compliance with vaccination scheme is greater when the program is mandatory, rather than voluntary; it is also known that when the employer pays for the vaccinations, compliance is markedly higher than if the employee must pay all or part of their immunization costs *(Miller and Palenik, 1998)*.

DHCP are at risk for exposure to, and possible infection with, infectious organisms. Immunizations substantially reduce both the number of (DHCP) susceptible to these diseases and the potential for disease transmission to other (DHCP) and patients *(Bolyard et al, 1998 and CDC, 1997)*. Thus, immunizations are an essential part of prevention and infection-control programs for (DHCP), and a comprehensive immunization policy should be implemented for all dental health-care facilities *(Association for Professionals in Infection Control and Epidemiology, 1999)*.

OSHA recommended that all health care workers with potential for exposure be offered the (HBV) vaccination at no cost to any (HCW) with reasonably anticipated exposure to blood *(Mahoney et al, 1997)*.

Fortunately, for dental professionals a vaccine has been developed to immunize against (HBV). Three doses are given to confer immunity: an initial dose, followed by a second dose at 1 month, and then a third dose 6 months after the first. Dental professionals are high risk of contracting (HBV), so that it is strongly recommended that all dental professionals should be obligatory immunized *(Gluck and Morganstein, 2003)*. Vaccine-induced antibodies decline gradually over time, and 60% of persons who initially respond to vaccination will lose detectable antibodies over 12 years *(CDC, 1997)*.

The Center for disease control and prevention (CDC) suggests that the limited number of reports of HBV transmission from health care workers to patients in recent years may reflect the adoption of standard precautions, and the increase in the use of hepatitis B vaccine *(Centers for Disease Control and Prevention, 2003)*.

I) Immunizations Strongly Recommended for (HCP):

As mentioned by *(CDC, 1997and Centers for Disease Control and Prevention, 2003)*;

Vaccine	Dose schedule
Hepatitis B Recombinant Vaccine	Three-dose schedule administered intramuscularly (IM) in the deltoid : 0,1,6–second dose administered 1 month after first dose: third dose administered 4 months after second. booster doses are not necessary for persons who have developed adequate antibodies to hepatitis B surface antigen (anti–HBs)
Influenza Vaccine (inactivated)	Annual single-dose vaccination IM with current vaccine.
Measles live - Virus vaccine	One dose administered Subcut-aneously (sc): second Dose ≥ 4 weeks later.
Mumps live - Virus vaccine	One dose SC: no booster.
Rubella live- Virus vaccine	One dose SC: no booster.
Varicella -Zoster Live-Virus vaccine	Two 0.5 ml doses SC 4-8 weeks apart if aged ≥ 13 years .

C) Effective training for staff:

Good training for all staff engaged in patient care is an important element of infection control. IC procedures should become an automatic part of clinical practices for all health care workers *(Wray et al, 2003)*.

Education and training should be appropriate to the assigned duties of specific (DHCP), e.g. techniques to prevent cross-contamination or instrument sterilization *(Bolyard et al ,1998 and US Department of Labor, Occupational Safety and Health Administration, 2001)*.

Each department in the hospital must have written polices and procedures for the control of infection. Caregivers and support personnel such as housekeepers and transport personnel must have periodic educational update on (IC) *(Craven and Hirnle, 2007)*.

Each practice must have a written (IC) policy. The policy should describe the practice policy for all aspects of (IC) and provide a useful guide to the training necessary for each member of staff to be competent and confident in its implementation. All members of the dental team must know who is responsible for ensuring certain activities and how they are carried out and to whom *(British Dental Association Advisory Service, 2003)*.

D) Needle Stick precaution:

Centers for Disease Control and Prevention (2001) mentioned that needle stick injuries and other percutaneous injuries are major occupational risks to health care workers. The results of the present study are similar to CDC. National Surveillances of Occupational Injuries for dental health care workers between 1995 and 2000 confirm that 44% of injuries were among dentists; meanwhile 19% of injuries were among dental assistants *(Gluck and Morganstein, 2003)*. Similar findings are mentioned by *(Dement et al, 2004)*: approximately 600,000 to 800,000 needle stick injuries occur annually in the United States healthcare hospital settings with estimation of 385,000 injuries to hospital based workers *(Gerberding, 2003)*. *Rogers, 2003* stated that 800,000 needle stick injures occur among health care workers each year in the United States, with half of the injures to nurses. Still, needle stick injures are seriously underreported, with underreporting rates range between 40% and 53% for nurses, between 70% and 95% for physicians, and about 92% for laboratory personnel.

Gershon et al (2005) mentioned that work stress has been shown to be related to workplace exposures to injuries, so that safe work behaviors are recommended. higher level of recapping needles of local anesthesia for tooth extraction among nurses, using wrong techniques of recapping with both hands, and work stress. Among dentists, the highest level of needles stick injury attributed to the support of gingival during injection of local anesthesia and unexpected patient movement: the patient may change his position as a response to pain, multiple injections of local anesthetic that may be required for one patient, or may be due to poor handling techniques form both nurses and dentists, or may be due to workload.

Needle stick injures predispose health team to the exposure to blood borne pathogens. Most such injures occur from attempt to recap the needle after use. Guidelines prohibit the recapping of needle and instruct the nurses to immediately dispose of sharps in puncture proof disposal containers, which must be carried at all times; when the sharp container become more than two -thirds full it should be disposed of appropriately according to agency protocol *(Mc Neal, 2000)*.

The most important behavioral risk factor for the transmission of (HCV) in developed countries became needle sharing and equipment sharing in the process of drug injection *(Alter, 1999)*.

Handling needles and sharp instruments like scalpels and scalers must be very careful because they easily puncture gloves and injure skin. Recap needles using a safe method or set them in a safe place without recapping them. If recapping, do not hold the cap with your hand, use a recapping device or "scoop up" the cap without touching it. One safe recapping method uses forceps to steady the cap. Never leave an uncapped needle on the treatment tray, because it is more likely to cause injury. Place it in a "sterile field" away from the bracket table until the procedure is complete *(Oeding and Mennito, 2005)*.

Several studies identified that clinical staff continued to recap needles without protection before disposing of the needles *(Scheutz and*

Langebaek, 1995). Precautions can be taken against occupational injuries but they are not completely controllable *(Wood, 1995)*.

E) Engineering controls:

Engineering controls are devices or equipments that reduce or eliminate a hazard. In the context of health care, this usually refers to device that provide protective guarding of sharp instruments such as needle or scalpel; devices that replace sharp items, such as needles with system that contain a sharp surfaces; and devices that eliminate worker exposure to sharp item, examples include sharps containers or needles covers with-built in retraction *(Draby and Walsh, 2003)*.

Occupational exposure is defined as reasonably anticipated skin, eye, mucous membrane, or parenteral contact with blood or other potentially infectious materials that can result from the performance of an employee's duties *(Centers for Disease Control and Prevention, 2003)*.

Engineering controls are designed to reduce employee exposure in the workplace by either removing or isolating the hazard or isolating the work from exposure. Self - sheathing needles, puncture - resistant containers are examples of engineering controls *(Rogers, 2003)*.

For blood borne pathogens, engineering controls that eliminate or isolate the hazard (e.g., puncture-resistant sharps containers or needle-retraction devices) are the primary strategies for protecting (DHCP) and patients. Where engineering controls are not available or appropriate, work-practice controls that result in safer behaviors (e.g., one-hand needle recapping or not using fingers for cheek retraction while using sharp instruments or suturing), and use of personal protective equipment (PPE) (e.g., protective eyewear, gloves, and mask) can prevent exposure *(Occupational Safety and Health Administration, 2001)*.

F) Principle guiding the management of sharps injuries:

(Samarnayake et al, 2002) stated the following action can be taken to manage sharps injuries:

1) First aids:

Wash puncture site thoroughly with soap and warm water; antiseptics may be used in addition, encourage bleeding by squeezing the injured area, and dry aseptically and report supervisor according to local regulations.

2) Future action:

Review hepatitis B, C, and HIV risk of source patients, inform source patients of the incident and counsel patients regarding HIV test, if indicated, and contact occupational Health Authority, as per local regulations.

3) Action by Occupational Health Authority:

Record in detail circumstance of the sharp injury (i.e. demographic information of the exposed worker, details of the exposure), check hepatitis B vaccination status of staff, if unvaccinated, and commence immediately hepatitis B vaccination procedures together with intramuscular hepatitis B immunoglobulin. Offer counseling to the recipient with regard to HIV risk. Arrange follow -up antibody testing at 6 months, or earlier if the recipient is anxious, and return details to Occupational Health Authority and the infection control team as appropriate.

G) Hand washing:

Hand washing is the most basic and effective infection control measure that prevents and controls the transmission of infectious agents *(Center for Diseases Control and prevention, 2000)*. Hand washing is an important and effective method in preventing the spread of infectious organism from one person to another *(Mailk, 2002)*.

Many infections result from cross transmission, primarily via the hands of health care workers (HCWs), so hand washing remains the single most important means to prevent the transmission of pathogens *(Pittet et al, 1999 and Boyce and Pittet , 2002)*.

Some microorganisms reside on the human body as normal flora, there are two type of normal flora: resident and transient. Resident flora are micro organisms that are always present, usually without altering the client health, considerable friction which is created by rubbing the hand and scribing the nails. Transient flora is episodic microorganisms for a brief period of time but do not continuously live on skin. Hand washing with soap and water is an effective mean for removing transient flora *(Daniels, 2004)*.

Hand washing, hand antisepsis, or surgical hand antisepsis, substantially reduces potential pathogens on the hands and is considered the single most critical measure for reducing the risk of transmitting organisms to patients and HCP *(CDC, 2002)*. Effective hand washing is recognized as one of the best means for preventing the spread of infections in hospitals *(Michaels et al, 2001)*. The aim of the procedure is to minimize potential for infection to patients, directly or indirectly, by hand contact to prevent health care personnel from becoming vectors of nosocomial pathogens *(Larson et al, 2000)*.

Hand washing is indicated before and after patient care, at any time hands become contaminated (even if gloved), hand washing with plain soap is adequate for examination and non surgical procedures. Antimicrobial surgical hand scrubbing is necessary with surgical procedures *(Gluck and Morganstein , 2003)*.

Any cuts or open skin lesions should be covered with a waterproof dressing. Dental health care workers who have exudative lesions or weeping dermatitis of the lower arms/hands or face, should refrain from direct patient contact until the condition is resolved *(NZDA, 2002)*.

Hand washing procedures

(Daniels, 2004) mentioned the following procedure should be implemented during hand washing:

1.   Remove jewelry. Wristwatch may be pushed up above the wrist (midforearm). Push sleeves of uniform or shirt up above the wrist at midforearm level.

2.   Assess hands for hangnails, cuts, or breaks in the skin, and areas that are heavily soiled.

3.   Turn on the water. Adjust the flow and temperature. Temperature of the water should be warm.

4.   Wet hands and lower forearms thoroughly by holding under running water. Keep hands and forearms in the down position with elbows straight. Avoid splashing water and touching the sides of the sink.

5.   Apply about 5 ml (1 teaspoon) of liquid soap. Lather thoroughly.

6.   Thoroughly rub hands together for about 10 to 15 seconds. Interlace fingers and thumbs and move back and forth to wash between digits. Rub palms and back of hands with circular

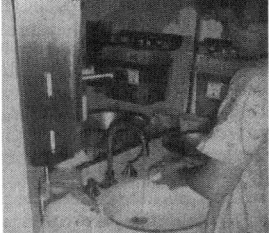 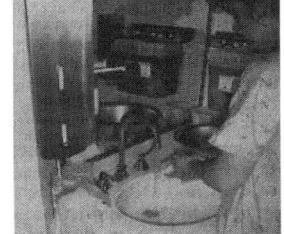

Figure (2): **lather thoroughly, and hands together.**

Figure (3): **Give special attention to finger nails and knuckles.**

(Cited from Daniels, 2004).

Nursing and the challenges toward implementing infection control strategies

7.   Special attention should be provided to areas such as the knuckles and fingernails, which are known to harbor organisms (figure 3).

8.   Rinse with hands in the down position, elbows straight. Rinse in the direction of forearm to wrist to fingers.

9.   Blot hands and forearms to dry thoroughly. Dry in the direction of fingers to wrist and forearms. Discard the paper towels in the proper receptacle.

10.   Turn off the water faucet with a clean, dry paper towel.

H) Personal Hygiene:

The whole dental team should be very careful about their personal hygiene. The staff should wear clean, fresh uniforms every day. Wash uniforms in hot soapy water and bleach. Machine dry at least at 100°F *(Oeding and Mennito, 2005)*.

Remove all jewelry before washing hands (including wedding rings) because soaps and chemicals can build up under rings and irritate your hands. Cover watches completely with gloves or long sleeves. Do not wear bracelets or earrings because they can become contaminated. Pull longer hair back away from the face. False fingernails can lift at the edge, creating an area for fungi and microorganisms to breed. Keep fingernails trimmed so they do not stress or puncture gloves. Keep cuts and sores always covered, not just when treating patients. Do not touch your face, nose, or mouth with contaminated gloves *(Oeding and Mennito, 2005)*.

I) Personal protective equipments:

Physical barriers play an important role in reducing cross-contamination and cross-infection between dental health care workers and their patients *(Wilson and Kornman, 2003)*.

Personal protective equipments should be used by health care workers who provide direct care to patients *(WHO, 2003)*.

The most important measure to minimize diseases transmission between patients and dental care providers is the routine use of gloves. All persons having direct patient contact should wear disposable gloves, disposable mask, gown and protective eye wear which should be worn during clinical dental procedure *(Phoenix et al, 2003)*.

I-1) Gloves:

Gloves protect dental team members from direct contact with microorganisms in patients' mouths and on contaminated surfaces and they also protect patients from microorganisms on the hand of the dental team *(Miller and Palenik, 1998)*.

All dentists and close support personnel should routinely wear disposable latex or vinyl gloves. A new pair of gloves should be worn for each patient , gloves should never reused and should be removed as soon as patient contact is over; face mask should not be touched with gloves during treatment *(Samarnayake et al, 2002)*.

DHCP should wear gloves to prevent contamination of their hands when touching mucous membranes, blood, saliva, or other potentially infectious materials and also to reduce the likelihood that microorganisms present on the hands of DHCP will be transmitted to patients during surgical or other patient care procedures *(Centers for Disease Control and Prevention, 2003)*.

Wearing gloves does not eliminate the need for hand washing. Hand hygiene should be performed immediately before wearing gloves. Gloves can have small, unapparent defects or can be torn during use, and hands can become contaminated during glove removal *(Murray et al, 2001)*.

Although the effectiveness of wearing two pairs of gloves in preventing disease transmission has not been demonstrated, the majority of studies among HCP and DHCP have demonstrated a lower frequency of inner glove perforation and visible blood on the surgeon's hands when double gloves are worn *(Avery et al, 1998)*.

Gloving procedures:

(Daniels, 2004) mentioned the following procedure should be implemented gloving procedures:

1. Wash hands.

2. Read the manufacturer's instructions on the package of sterile gloves; proceed as directed in removing the outer wrapper from the package (figure4 and 5) and in placing the inner wrapper

onto a clean, dry surface (figure 6). Open inner wrapper to expose gloves (figure 7).

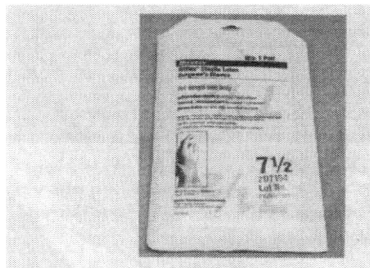

Figure (4): Sterile glove

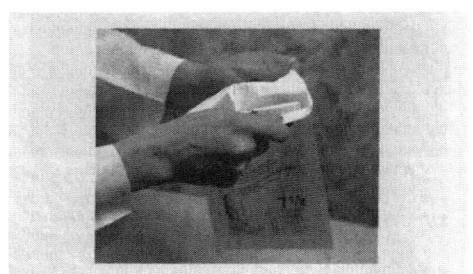

Figure (5): **Remove the outer wrapper of the sterile glove package**

(Cited from Daniels, 2004).

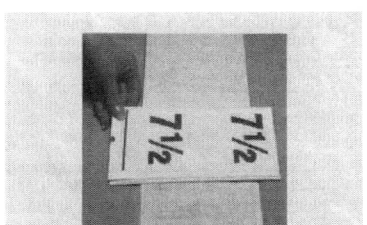

Figure (6): **Place the gloves in the inner wrapper on clean, dry surface**

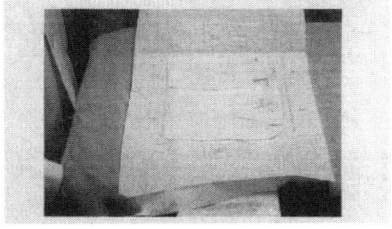

Figure (7): **Open the inner wrapper to expose gloves**

(Cited from Daniels, 2004).

3. Identify right and left hand; glove dominant hand first.

4. Grasp the 2-inch- (5-cm) wide cuff with the thumb and first two fingers of the nondominant hand, touching only the cuff (figure 8).

Nursing and the challenges toward implementing infection control strategies

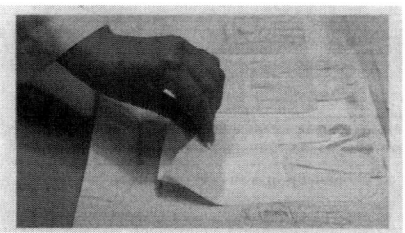

Figure (8): **Grasp first cuff with the nondominant hand**

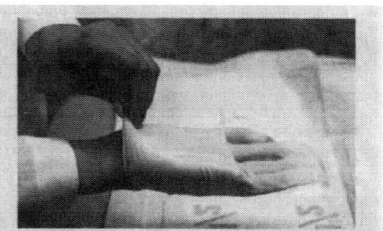

Figure (9): **Pull the glove over the dominant hand.**

(Cited from Daniels, 2004).

5.   Gently pull the glove over the dominant hand, making sure the thumb and fingers fit into the proper spaces of the glove (figure 9). Hold hands above the waist while applying glove. Once dominant hand is gloved, keep hands visible and above waist to prevent accidental contamination.

6.   With the gloved dominant hand, slip your fingers under the cuff of the other glove, gloved thumb abducted, making sure it does not touch any part on your nondominant hand (figure 10). Be careful not to drag glove or touch gloved dominant hand with ungloved nondominant hand.

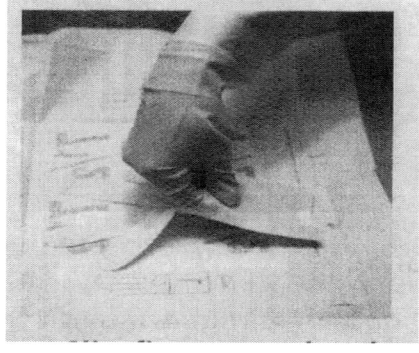

Figure (10): Slip fingers under the cuff of the second glove.

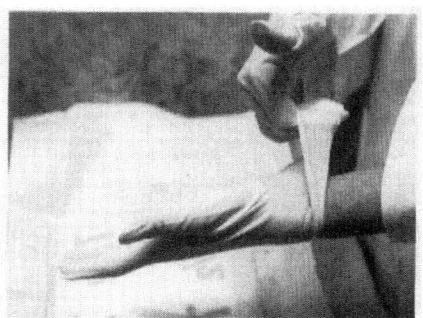 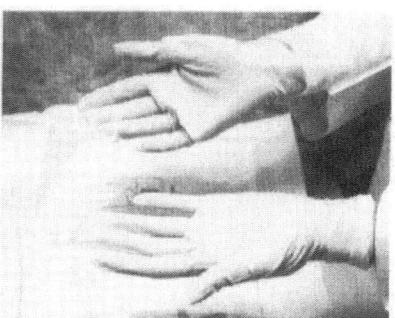

Figure (11): **Pull on the second glove**

Figure (12): **Make sure all fingers are in the proper space**

7. With gloved hands, interlock fingers to fit the gloves onto each finger.

8. Slip gloved fingers of the dominant hand under the cuff of the opposite hand, or grasp the outer part of the glove at the wrist if there is no cuff.

9. Pull the glove down to the fingers, exposing the thumb.

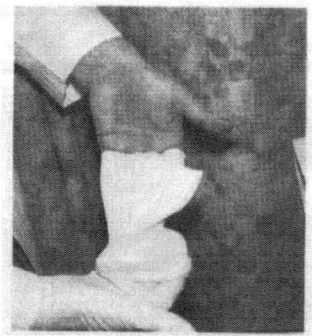

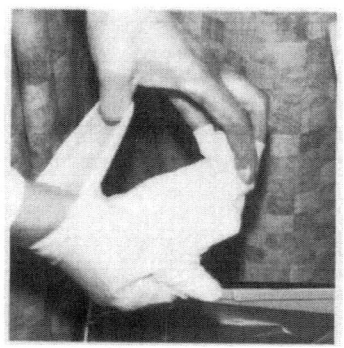

Figure (13): Peel glove down to
fingers, exposing one thump.

Figure (14): Slip uncovered thumb
into the opposite glove.

(Cited from Daniels, 2004).

10. Slip the uncovered thumb into the opposite glove at the wrist, allowing only the glove-covered fingers of the hand to touch the solied glove.

11. Pull the glove down over the dominant hand almost to the fingertips, and slip the glove on to the other hand.

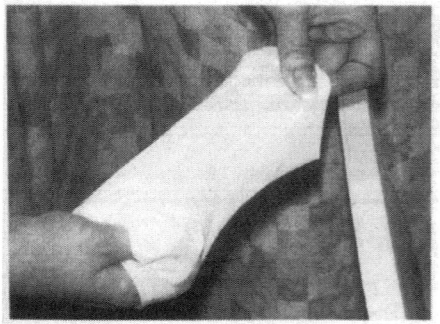

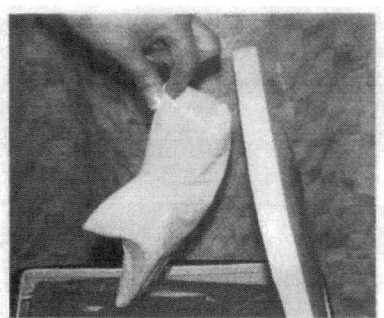

Figure (15): When soled gloves are removed
correctly, only the inside clean surface of one
glove is exposed.

Figure (16): Dispose of gloves in
appropriate receptacle.

Nursing and the challenges toward implementing infection control strategies

12. With the dominant hand touching only the inside of the other glove, pull the glove over the dominant hand so that only the inside (clean surface) is exposed.

13. Dispose of soiled gloves according to institutional policy and wash hands.

I-2) Eye protection:

In the course of many dental procedures, body fluids of the patients may be presented in the splash or spray from dental devices. Additionally, blood or saliva may be present in particles generated and released during the procedures. The DHCW performing, assisting or closely observing procedure where it is reasonable to suspect that droplet, aerosol or particles may be produced must wear protective eye wear *(Silverman et al, 2001)*.

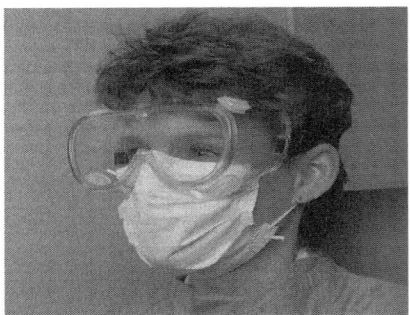

Figure (17): **Nurse wearing protective goggles and mask.**
Cited from (Potter, and Perry, 2001).

Nursing and the challenges toward implementing infection control strategies

I-3) Mask:

Masks should be worn under the same circumstances that warrant the use of eye protection *(Draby and Walsh, 2003)*.

Surgical and procedure masks are adequate during most dental procedure to protect the nose, mouth and airway from contact with body fluids. A new mask should be used for each patient *(Silverman et al, 2001)*.

The mask's outer surface can become contaminated with infectious droplets from spray of oral fluids or from touching the mask with contaminated fingers; also when a mask becomes wet from exhaled moist air, the resistance to airflow through the mask increases, causing more airflow to pass around edges of the mask. If the mask becomes wet, it should be changed between patients or even during patient treatment when possible *(CDC, National Institute for Occupational Safety and Health, 1999)*.

Procedures guidelines for wearing mask:

(Potter, and Perry, 2001) mentioned the following procedures for wearing mask :

1. Find top edge of mask (usually has thin metal strip along edge.). pliable metal fits snugly against bridge of nose.

2. Hold mask by top two strings or loops. Ti two top ties at top of back of head (see illustration), with ties above ears. (Alternative: Slip loops over each ear).

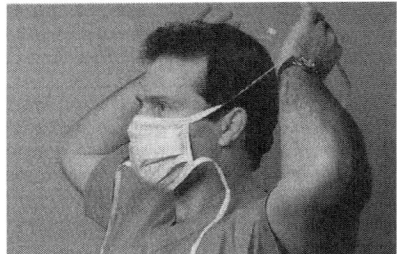

Figure (18): **Hold mask by top two strings or loops**

3. Tie two lower ties snugly around neck with mask well under chin (see illustration).

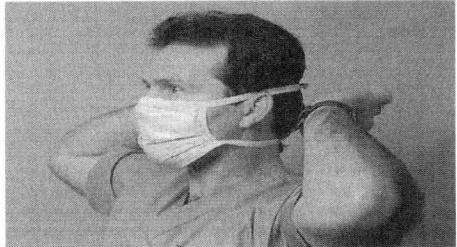

Figure (19): **Tie two lower ties snugly around neck with mask well under chin**

Cited from (Potter, and Perry, 2001).

Nursing and the challenges toward implementing infection control strategies

4.   Gently pinch upper metal band around bridge of nose.

Note: Mask should be changed if wet, moist, or contaminated.

I-4) Protective clothing:

Attire that prevents the contact of blood; other bodily fluids, secretions, and execration with work clothes, street clothes, and skin. For most dental procedures, a gown or lab coat with long sleeves and collar sufficient to cover exposed clothing and skin. Surgical Procedures may require the use of attire made from material with fluid resistant properties. Disposable gowns are also acceptable as long they meet the criteria for barrier protection *(Silverman et al, 2001)*.

DHCP should change protective clothing daily or between patients if it has become visibly soiled, and as soon as it is feasibly penetrated by blood or other potentially infectious fluid. All protective clothing should be removed before leaving the work area *(US Department of Labor, Occupational Safety and Health Administration, 2001)*.

Personnel may wear a specific uniform. A clean and freshly laundered uniform should be worn each day/duty. The uniform can be domestically laundered. Food and drink must not be consumed in the clinical and sterilizing areas *(NZDA, 2002)*.

Steps for applying gown :

(Potter, and Perry, 2001) mentioned the following procedure should be implemented for applying gown:

1. Before entering operating room or treatment area, apply cap, face mask, and eyewear. Foot covers are also required in operating room.

2. Perform thorough hand wash.

3. Ask circulating nurse to assist by opening sterile pack containing sterile gown (folded inside out).

4. Have circulation nurse prepare glove package by peeling outer wrapper open while keeping inner contents sterile. Inner glove package is then placed on sterile field created b sterile outer wrapper.

5. Reach down sterile gown package (see illustration); lift folded gown directly upward and step back away from table (see illustration).

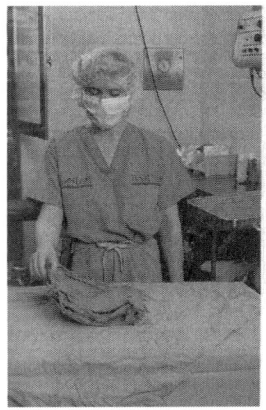 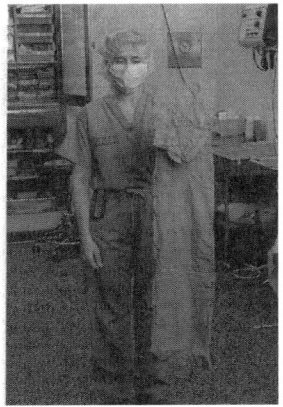

Figure (20): **Reach sterile gown package**   *Cited from (Potter, and Perry, 2001).*

Nursing and the challenges toward implementing infection control strategies

6.   Holding folded gown, locate neckband. With both hands, grasp inside front of gown just below neckband (see illustration).

7.   Allow gown to unfold, keeping inside of gown toward body. Do not touch outside of gown with bare hands (see illustration).

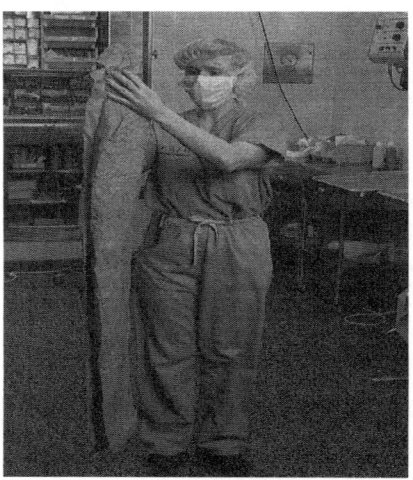

Figure (21): **Allow gown to unfold, keeping inside of gown toward body**
Cited from (Potter, and Perry, 2001).

8.   With hands at shoulder level, slip both arms into armholes simultaneously (see illustration). Ask circulating nurse to bring gown over shoulders by reaching inside to arm seams. Gown is pulled on, leaving sleeves covering hands (see illustration).

9.   Have circulating nurse securely tie back of gown at neck and waist. (If gown is a wraparound style, sterile flap to cover gown is not touched until the nurse has gloved).

Nursing and the challenges toward implementing infection control strategies

Closed Gloving:

1. With hands covered by gown sleeves, open inner sterile glove package.

2. With nondominant hand inside gown cuff, pick up glove for dominant hand by grasping folded cuff.

3. Extend dominant forearm with palm up and place palm of glove against palm of dominant hand. Glove fingers will point toward elbow.

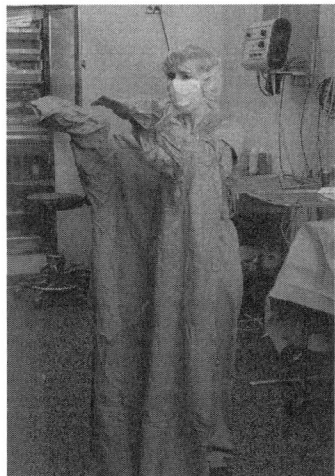 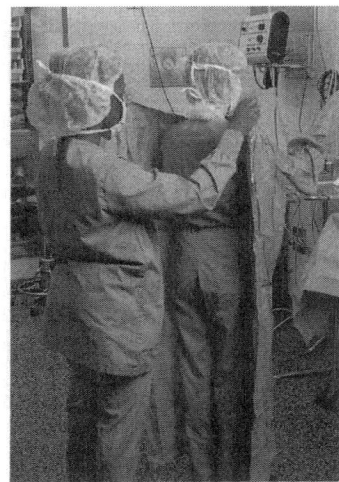

Figure (22): **For wraparound sterile gowns**

Cited from (Potter, and Perry, 2001).

4. Grasp back of glove cuff with nondominant hand and turn glove cuff over end of dominant hand and gown cuff (see illustration).

Nursing and the challenges toward implementing infection control strategies

5. Grasp top of glove and underlying gown sleeve with covered nondominant hand. Carefully extend fingers into glove, being sure glove's cuff gown's cuff.

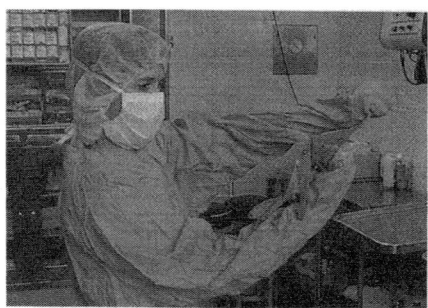

Figure (23): **Grasp back of glove cuff with nondominant hand and turn glove cuff over end of dominant hand and gown cuff**

Cited from (Potter, and Perry, 2001).

6. Glove nondominant hand in same manner, reversing hands (see illustration). Use gloved dominant hand to pull on glove. Keep hand sleeve (see illustration).

7. Be sure fingers are fully extended into both gloves.

8. For wraparound sterile gowns: take gloved hand and release fastener or ties in front of gown.

9. Hand tie to sterile team member who stands still. Allowing margin of safety, turn around to the left, covering back with extended gown flap. Take back tie from team member and secure tie to gown.

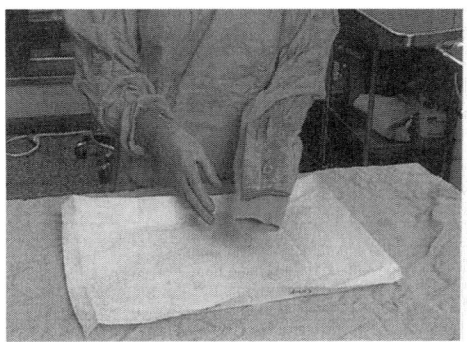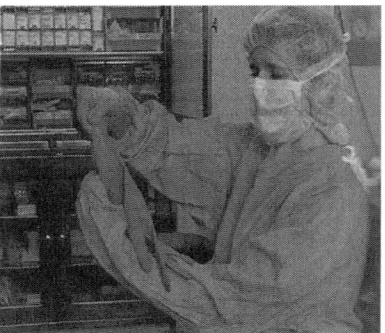

Figure (24): **Glove nondominant hand in same manner**

Cited from (Potter, and Perry, 2001).

J) Use of disposables instruments and equipments:

The best way to control cross- contamination is to use disposables. The following disposable article are available in dentistry: Needles, syringes, rubber cups, surfaces covers, gloves, masks gown, saliva ejector tips, head cap for surgeons and the patients patient napkin, and suction tips *(Chandra et al, 2002)*. Disposable items are recommended; although there is a cost implication, disposable items must always be used once only and then discarded *(Wray et al, 2003)*.

Use a new, sterile disposable needle for every patient requiring local anesthesia, and never reuse needles for different patients *(Oeding and Mennito, 2005)*.

K) Protection against aerosols and spatter:

Spray and spatter from the patient's mouth must be reduced to minimum to reduce contamination; so that high power suction must be used for this purpose *(Chandra et al, 2002)*.

L) Instruments preparation:

Instruments to be heat sterilized should be cleaned by scrubbing with hot water and soap or by using an ultrasonic cleaner. Instruments should then be dried, packed, and heat sterilized *(Phoenix et al, 2003)*.

Ultrasonic cleaner which is many times more effective and safer than hand scrubbing, should be the choice for definitive instrument cleaning. Dental staff performing such procedures of cleaning and packing of contaminated instruments should wear reusable, heavy rubber work gloves similar to household gloves. Contaminated instruments that will not be cleaned immediately should be submersed in holding solution so that blood, saliva, and tissues will not dry on the instrument surfaces *(Cohen and Burns, 2002)*.

M) Decontamination, disinfection and sterilization of instruments:

Decontamination: means the cleaning - either through manual or mechanical method of visible dirt or bioburden. Decontamination must occur prior to disinfection or sterilization procedures *(NZDA, 2002)*.

Decontamination is the combination of processes (including cleaning, disinfection and sterilization) used to make a reusable item safe for further use on patients and handling by staff *(NHS, 2000)*.

Disinfection is defined as: Destruction of pathogenic and other kinds of microorganisms by physical or chemical means. Disinfection is less lethal than sterilization, because it destroys the majority of recognized pathogenic microorganisms, but not necessarily all microbial forms (e.g., bacterial spores). Disinfection does not ensure the degree of safety associated with sterilization processes *(Centers for Disease Control and Prevention, 2003)*.

Disinfection refers to the elimination of most harmful bacteria from an article so as to render it safe for use (Mahon and Sloan, 2000). Disinfection must never be used when sterilization is possible *(Arora and Arora, 2003)*.

Sterilization is defined as the process by which an article, a surface or a medium is freed of all microorganisms including viruses' bacteria, their spores and fungi both pathogenic and non pathogenic *(Arora and Arora, 2003)*.

The best and safest approach to preventing disease transmission from patient to patient via the instruments is to sterilize all reusable instruments that are contaminated with blood or saliva instead of sterilizing some and disinfecting others. Sterilizers must be used correctly to achieve sterilization *(Oeding and Mennito, 2005)*. Sterilization of medical and dental instruments is fundamental to infection control in health care settings *(Acosta-Gío et al, 2002)*.

Dental practice by unregistered practitioners is common in developing countries; besides their technical incompetence, they do not properly sterilize their equipments and thereby transmit blood borne infections to their patients. Strict enforcement of legislation to ban such illegal practices may result in substantial reduction in HBV transmission in this and similar settings *(Akhtar et al, 2005)*.

Much of the equipments in the dental department are not used in the mouth, is straightforward to decontaminate using well-established principles and methods *(British Dental Association Advisory Service, 2003 and Centers for Disease Control, 1993)*. Many intra-oral items are available for single patient use and are then immediately disposed of as clinical waste ,for example hypodermic needles, cotton wool plugs *(Weightman and Lines, 2004)*.

Reprocessing of instruments used in dental practices should follow the classification of critical (used to penetrate soft tissue or bone and require sterilization), semi critical (do not penetrate, but have contact with oral tissues and should be sterilized if capable of withstanding the process or undergo high level disinfection), and non critical (contact skin and require intermediate level or low-level disinfection). Appropriate cleaning and use of appropriate personal protective equipment during reprocessing are necessary *(USPHS, DHHS, and Centers for Disease Control and Prevention, 2003)*.

Nursing and the challenges toward implementing infection control strategies

Sterilization of all instruments that can withstand heat sterilization must be cleaned and heat sterilized between the uses of chemical disinfection of these items is unacceptable *(Phoenix et al, 2003)*.

Sterilization methods:

The most important methods for sterilization are the following:

1. ***Steam autoclave:*** it used at 121^0C for 15-20 min, it have many advantages such as, it short cycle method, good penetration material compatibility, and from the disadvantages, carbon steel correction, dulling of cutting edges, and wet packaging *(Silverman et al, 2001)*.

2. ***Dry heat:*** it used at 160 0C for 2 hr or 170 0C for 1 hr is advantages, effective and safe method cause no dulling, no rust/correction. On other hand it is long cycle, poor penetration, not used for sterilizing dental handpices *(Silverman et al , 2001)*.

3. ***Chemical:*** are effective disinfectant because they attack all types of microorganisms, act rapidly, work with water, retain no order are stable in light and heat , inexpensive, are not harmful to body tissues, don't destroy articles being disinfected and are not inactivated by organic material *(Potter and Perry, 2001)*.

4. ***Gas:*** such as Ethylene Oxide, this gas destroys spores microorganisms by altering cell metabolic processes, fumes are realized within autoclave realized chamber. Ethylene Oxide gas

is toxic to humans and aeration time various within product, this gas sterilize some rubber and plastic items *(Potter and Perry, 2001)*.

5. ***Radiation:*** ionizing radiation penetrates deeply in to objects for effective sterilization and disinfection, it used for sterilizing drugs, food and other heat sensitive items *(Potter and Perry, 2001)*.

N) Cleaning and disinfection of environmental surfaces:

Surfaces most likely to become contaminated with bioburden (body fluid/spoilage/splatter) as a result of treatment procedures are to be cleaned and then disinfected after each patient consultation. These surfaces include, but are not limited to the patient chair, dental tray, spittoon, overhead light handle, x-ray head and any items/surfaces which have been contaminated with bioburden from dental personnel gloves. Disposable contact wrap or commercially available covers, where applicable, can be used on frequently contaminated surfaces, eliminating the need for cleaning/disinfecting. The wrap/cover must be changed between patients *(NZDA, 2002)*.

Contamination of hand contact surfaces might be implicated in the spread of micro-organisms within hospitals, could act as a reservoir for microorganisms, and could contribute to hand contamination during or after hand washing. In addition, a number of organic soils on surfaces have been found to provide protective effects furthering the survival of potential pathogens *(Moore and Griffith, 2001)*.

O) Disposal of wastes:

Hospitals have the responsibility to ensure safe disposal of contaminated waste. Arrangement must be made with a local authority; all sharp items must be consigned to rigid puncture resistant containers, never to be filled to more than two thirds of their capacity. The containers should be securely closed and fastened before uplift for incineration. Soft waste contaminated with blood must be placed into sturdy, impervious, sealed bags and clearly labeled as infective waste *(Wray et al, 2003)*.

Incineration:

Incineration is a method of soiled and hazardous waste managements. Incineration reduces the volume of wastes by up to 90% and is effective in destroying most biological contaminants. However, increasing air pollution, particularly with toxic chemicals and subsequent disposal process for residual heavy metal are the primary concern *(Mc Ewen, 2002)*. Incineration should be installed at appropriate location to avoid nuisance to patients and neighborhood .Infected waste can be incinerated, put in a deep landfill or be made part of the municipal collection system after treatments with a disinfection for 30 minutes. However, needles, syringes, and other infected sharp wastes should be destroyed mechanically *(Arora and Arora, 2003)*.

P) Role of the nurse in infection control measures :

Community health nurse role varies according to each client's needs and from setting to setting, and there is universal nursing intervention and roles that are required of virtually all nurses in almost all settings *(Mc closkey and Bulecken, 2000)*.

- *For example*, **infection control:** minimizing the acquisition and transmission of infectious agents.
- **Environmental managements (safety):** monitoring and manipulation of the physical environment to promote safety *(MC Ewen, 2002)*.

The nurse plays a critical role in minimizing infection spread by understanding the chain of infection, the nurse can intervene to prevent infection from developing, by minimizing number and kinds of organisms transmitted to potential infection site, proper cleaning, disinfection and sterilization of contaminated objectives significantly reduce and often eliminate microorganisms. Eliminating reservoirs of infection, controlling portal of exit and entry, and avoiding actions that transmit microorganisms prevent infection from finding a new site in which to grow. Proper use of sterile supplies, barriers protection and proper hand washing are examples of the methods that a nurse must use to control the spread of microorganisms. Having an (IC) conscience helps the nurse to apply good aseptic practices at the right time and right clinical situation. When a client has an infection, the nurse continues preventive care so that health care personnel and other clients are not exposed to infection *(Potter and Perry, 2001)*.

Community health nurse who provide quality care must have basic understanding of epidemiology, infection control, microbiology, medicine, and public health nursing. Furthermore, the community nurse must have knowledge of the legal system which mandate prevention and control of communicable diseases locally, nationally, and worldwide *(Smitch and Maurer, 1995)*.

The (IC) procedures must be followed to eliminate pathway of cross- contamination from patient to dental team and from dental team to patients are: wear gloves, mask, protective clothing, eyewear, hand washing, wear heavy gloves for clean-up, ultrasonic cleaning rather than hand-scribing, instrument cassettes to reduce direct handling during cleaning, surfaces disinfection, immunization, instrument sterilization, needle safety and waste managements *(Miller and Palenik, 1998)*.

To eliminate pathway of cross -contamination from patient to patient, the following procedure must be followed: instrument sterilization, monitoring of sterilization, hand washing, proper gloving, change of masks, change of protective clothing when needed, decontaminate protective eyewear, surfaces disinfection, surfaces covering, and the use of sterile or clean supplies *(Miller and Palenik, 1998)*.

Pathway of cross -contamination from dental office to community can be eliminated through: waste management and proper management of contaminated laundry. Immunization, and hand washing are key tools to eliminate infection to dental team family. To eliminate pathway of cross-contamination from community to patient; use of new and separate water source, periodically disinfect dental unit water line, using water containing antimicrobial agent, and filter the water *(Miller and Palenik, 1998)*.

To improve health care workers compliance with practices, infection control professionals should learn from the behavioral sciences. IC professionals play key roles in the identification and prevention of infections. They act as observers and educators and, ultimately, should become change agents. Changing behavior and shifting social norms at multiple levels through the health care worker community are among the key challenges of (IC) today *(Pittet, 2005)*.

The duties of the dental nurse range from assisting the dentist in clinical procedures to managing the practice *(John et al, 2002)*.

Control of infection is an important part of every action the nurse performs; the nurse's knowledge of infection, application of infection control principles and use of common sense help protect patients from infection. In many situations nurses are exposed to pathogenic microorganisms and should use both specialized and routine practices of cleanliness and disinfection to prevent the spread of infection *(Christensen, and Kockrow, 2006)*.

Dental nurses need to be aware of health and safety procedures with respect to the potentially hazardous materials and equipments that are used in the dental surgery. With the dangers of hepatitis and HIV infection, all dental personnel need to be trained in cross-infection control techniques. In dentistry requires assistance of a trained dental nurse familiar with clinical procedures for the safety of the patient *(John et al, 2002)*.

IC consists of polices and procedures of hospitals or other health care facility to minimize the risk of nosocomial or community - acquired infections spreading to patients and other staff members. IC is a routine whatever action a nurse performs *(Christensen, and Kockrow, 2006)*.

To minimize the risk of cross infection in the dental office, specific recommendations have been issued by professional health agencies. These recommendations include the routine use of barrier techniques (gloves, masks), heat sterilization of dental instruments, vaccination against HBV, and implementing the universal precautions *(Al-Omari and Dwairi, 2005)*.

Infection control nurse (ICN):

Many agencies employ nurses who are specially trained in (IC). They are responsible for advising hospital personnel on safe aseptic practices and for monitoring infection outbreak within the agency *(Christensen, and Kockrow, 2006)*.

ICN is the only member of the (IC) team with a full - time responsibility for (IC), enabling him or her to maintain a clinical input within ward and departments and always to be accessible for advice and support *(Ayliffe et al, 2000)*. She should responsible for (IC) in trust should be graded as a clinical nurse specialist or senior nurse manager and have access and links across all clinical directorates *(Ayliffe et al, 2000)*.

The attendance of ICNs at the annual conference in the field of IC should be considered as part of their training and mandatory *(Ayliffe et al, 2000)*.

ICN is a member of and share responsibility with the (IC) team, the nurse should visit all wards regularly and discuss any problems with the staff, the laboratory should be visit every morning by ICN. Instruction of nurses in the practices of infection control is one of the major responsibilities, and should be treated as a priority *(Ayliffe et al, 2000)*.

The day- to- day activates of ICN includes the following:

- Participation in teaching and practical demonstration of techniques for control of infection to medical, nursing, auxiliary and, other profession allied to medicine ;
- identifying as promptly as possible potential infection hazards in patients, staff or equipments;
- conferring with the sterile service manger about the management of equipment used by patients with certain infection e.g. hepatitis B virus;
- collaborating with and advising community nurse on problems of infection ;
- promptly supply information about notifiable diseases by telephone to the public health medical officer;
- informing other hospitals ,general practitioners and other health - care providers when infected patients are discharged or transferred to elsewhere, and receiving relevant information from other hospitals or from the community where appropriate;

- produce and update (IC) policies   and guidelines ;
- informing the director of nursing and/directorate nurse manager of practical problems and difficulties in carrying out routine procedures related to nursing aspect of (IC) ;
- offer advice on purchase and decontamination of equipments;
- regular audit of relevant wards in unit to ensure that infection control procedures are being carried out in accordance with hospital policy *(Ayliffe et al , 2000)*.

References

- *Abdel All, S.E.* (1998): Factors affecting nurses practices related to universal infection prevention control precautions in Heamodialysis Unit of Tanta University Hospital, Thesis, Faculty of Nursing, Alexandria University.

- *Abdullah, E.H.* (1996): The relation ship between the knowledge base of nursing staff and the quality of infection control at the Main University Hospital in Alexandria, Thesis, Faculty of Nursing, Alexandria University.

- *Abou Shadi, N., and Ibrahim, S*. (2001): Implementation and evaluation of educational program for nurses regarding nosocomial infection control at Mansoura University Hospital . The new Egyptian Journals of Medicine; 24(5) : 2226- 33.

- *Abo-zeid, H., A.* (2006):Assessment of knowledge practices and attitudes of workers in Assiut University toward elderly care, Thesis Master, Faculty of Nursing, Assiut University.

- *Acosta-Gío, A., Mata-Portuguez, V.H, Herrero-Farías A, and Pérez, L.S.* (2002): Biologic monitoring of dental office sterilizers in Mexico, AJIC 30 (3): 153 -157.

- *Acquired Immunodeficiency Syndrome "AIDS".* (1983): Precautions for health care workers and allied professionals, MMWR Morb Mortal Wkly Rep 32.

- *Agostinho, A.M, Miyoshi, P.R, Gnoatto N, Paranhos, H.O, de Figueired L.C, and Salvador L.S.* (2004): Cross-contamination in the dental laboratory through the polishing procedure of complete dentures, Braz. Dent. J. 15(2).

- *Ahmed, A.* (1996): Assessment of nurses' knowledge and practices regarding universal infection control precautions of blood borne pathogens. Unpublished Master thesis, Alexandria University, Faculty of Nursing.

- *Ajemian , E., and Castle, M.* (1987): Hospital infection control . 2nd ed., New York: Johnwilez and sons Inc., P. 1, 37.

- *Akhtar, S., Younus, M., Adil, S., Hassan, F., and Jafri, S.H.* (2005): Research article, Epidemiologic study of chronic hepatitis B virus infection in male volunteer blood donors in Karachi, Pakistan BMC Gastroenterology ; 5:5-26

- *Allender, J.A and Spradley, B.W.* (2001): Community Health Nursing Concept and practice. Communicable diseases control, 5th ed, Lippincott, Philadelphia, pp.298-309.

- *Al-Omari, M.A, and Dwairi, Z.N.* (2005): Compliance with Infection Control Programs in Private Dental Clinics in Jordan, J Dent Educ. 69(6) Pp. 693-698 .

- *Al-Rabeah, A., and Mohamed, A.G.* (2002): Infection Control In The Private Dental Sector In Riyadh, Annals of Saudi Medicine 22(1-2), Pp13-17.

- *Alter, M. J.* (1999): HCV infection in the United States. J. Hepatol. 31(Suppl.1):88-91.

- *American Dental Association,* (1996): Infection control recommendation in the dental office and dental laboratories. The Journals of the American Dental Association; 127(5):672- 680.

- *American Dental Association* (1998): Infection control recommendations for the dental office and dental laboratory. Journal of the American Dental Association, 116:241-8.

- *Andreoll T., Bennett, J., Carpenter., C.* (1998): Essential of Medicine. El sensory, T. Assessment of infection Prevention measures carried out in the surgical wards in different types of hospitals in Cairo, Review articles, Faculty of Nursing, Alexandria University, p 4.

- *Angelillo, I.F, Villari, P., D'Errico, M.M, Grasso, G.M, Ricciardi G., and Pavia, M.* (1994): Dentists and AIDS: a survey of knowledge, attitudes and behaviors in Italy. J Public Health Dent; 54, Pp145–52.

- *Arora, D.R, and Arora, H.* (2003): A textbook of Microbiology for Dental Students. Sterilization and Disinfection ,3rd ed ,CBS Publishers and Distributors, Darya Ganj, New Delhi ,Pp23 -32.

- *Arthur, R.R, Hassan, N.F, and Abdallah, M.Y, et al* (1997): Hepatitis C antibody prevalence in blood donors in different governorates in Egypt. Trans R Soc Trop Med Hyg91 pp: 271-274.

- *Association for Professionals in Infection Control and Epidemiology. APIC position paper* (1999): immunization. Am J Infect Control; 27:52-53.

- *Avery, C.M, Hjort, A., Walsh, S., and Johnson, P.A.* (1998): Glove perforation during surgical extraction of wisdom teeth. Oral Surg Oral Med Oral Pathol Oral Radiol Endod; 86:23-50.

- *Ayliffe G.A, Lawbury, E.J, Gerrds, A.M, Williams , J.D.* (1992): Control of hospital infection, 3rd ed., New York : Chapman and Hall Co., p.10.

- *Ayliffe, G.A, Fraise, A.P, Gaddes, A.M and Mitchell, L.K.* (2000): Control of hospital infection A practical hand book, Introduction, Administration and responsibility, 4th ed, Arnold, A member of the Hodder Head , London ,pp. 1-24.

- *Bagg, J., Sweeney, C.P, Roy, K.M, Sharp, T., and Smith, A.* (2002): Cross infection control measures and the treatment of patients at risk of Creutzfeldt Jakob Disease in UK general dental practice, British Dental Journal;191 (2), Pp.87-90.

- *Bahget, R.* (1999): Factors Affecting Nurses' Knowledge and Practices related to Universal Precaution for Infection Control in the premature Unit at Tanta Hospital. Journal of the Medical research Institutes; 20(2) :147-62.

- ***Bannister B.A, Begg, N.T, Gillespis, S.H.*** (2000): Infectious diseases. In Moustada, M.M. Nosocomial Infection. Review articles, Faculty of Nursing, Alexandria University; P.5.

- ***Beder, N.A, and Michel, H.W.*** (2004): Impact of Universal Infection Control Intervention Program for Nurses; 3(1):13-24.

- ***Bennett, J.V, and Brachman, P.H.S*** (1998): Hospital infection, 4th ed., Philadelphia: Lippincott. Raven Publishers. Pp.3- 4.

- ***Bentley, E.M, and Sarll, D.W.*** (1995): Improvements in cross-infection control in general dental practice. Br Dent J; 179: Pp.19-21.

- ***Berhe, M., Michael, B., Edmond, M., and Gonzalo, M.*** (2005): Practiceshttp://www.sciencedirect.com/science?_ob=ArticleURL&_udi=B6W9M-4FC3626-H&_user=1052409&_coverDate=02%2F01%2F2005&_alid=442900715&_rdoc=28&_fmt=full&_orig=search&_cdi=6686&_sort=d&_docanchor=&view=c&_acct=C000051060&_version=1&_urlVersion=0&_use and an assessment of health care workers' perceptions of compliance with infection control _knowledge of nosocomial infections, Am J Infect Control 33, Pp. 55-57.

- ***Bischoff, W.E, Reynolds, T.M, Cessler, C.N, Edmond, M.B, and Wenzel, R.P.*** (2000): Hand washing compliance by health care workers: the impact of introducing an accessible, alcohol-based hand antiseptic, Arch Intern Med 160, Pp. 1017–1021.

- ***Bolyard, E.A, Tablan, O.C, Williams, W.W, Pearson. M.L, Shapiro, C.N, and Deitchman, S.D.*** (1998): Hospital Infection Control

Nursing and the challenges toward implementing infection control strategies

Practices Advisory Committee. Guideline for infection control in health care personnel, 1998. Am J Infect Control; 26: pp.289-354.

- **_Boyce, J.M. and Pittet, D._** (2002): Healthcare Infection Control Practices Advisory Committee, HICPAC/SHEA/APIC/IDSA Hand Hygiene Task Force. Guideline for Hand Hygiene in Health-Care Settings. Recommendations of the Healthcare Infection Control Practices Advisory Committee and the HICPAC/SHEA/APIC/IDSA Hand Hygiene Task Force, MMWR 51 (RR-16), pp. 1– 45.

- **_Bray, S., and Chapman, S._** (1990): AIDS and dentistry in Australia: knowledge, infection control practices and attitudes to treatment in a 'random' sample of Australian dentists. Community Health Studies 14, Pp. 384–393.

- **_British Dental Association Advisory Service_** (2003): Infection control in dentistry. British Dental Association Advice Sheet A12. 'Pp1-21. http://www.udp.org.uk/resources/bda-cross-infection.pdf

- **_Burke,_** http://www.sciencedirect.com/science?_ob=ArticleURL&_udi=B6T86-44B85C8-1&_user=1052409&_coverDate=11%2F30%2F2001&_alid=441899575&_rdoc=3&_fmt=full&_orig=search&_cdi=5078&_sort=d&_docanchor=&view=c&_acct=C000051060&_version=1&_urlVersion=0&_user **_F.J.T, Wilson, N.H.F, Wastell, D.G. et al._** (1991): Glove use in clinical practice: a survey of 2000 dentists in England and Wales. British Dental Journal 171, Pp. 128–132.

- *Centers for Disease Control. Recommended infection-control practices for dentistry.* (1986): MMWR Morb Mortal Wkly Rev; 35:237–42.

- *Centers for Disease Control* (1993): Recommended infection control practices for dentistry. MMWR Morb Mortal Wkly Rep 42 RR-8; 35.pp .237-242.

- *CDC* (1997): Immunization of health-care workers, recommendations of the Advisory Committee on Immunization Practices (ACIP) and the Hospital Infection Control Practices Advisory Committee (HICPAC). MMWR; 46(No. RR-18).

- *CDC. National Institute for Occupational Safety and Health* (1999): TB respiratory protection program in health care facilities: administrator's guide. Cincinnati, OH: US Department of Health and Human Services, Public Health Service, CDC, National Institute for Occupational Safety and Health, DHHS publication no. (NIOSH) 99-143.

- *Center for Diseases Control and Prevention* (2000).CDC: Media Relation why is Hand washing important? http:// www.cdc.gov/ ncidod/nicd.htm.

- *Centers for Disease Control and Prevention* (2001): Updated U.S. Public Health Service Guidelines for management of occupational exposure to HBV, HCV, and HIV and recommendations for post-exposure prophylaxis. Atlanta (GA): Centers for Disease Control and Prevention Guidelines; 50 (RR-11).

- ***CDC*** (2002): Guideline for hand hygiene in health-care settings : recommendations of the Healthcare Infection Control Practices Advisory Committee and the HICPAC/SHEA/ APIC/ IDSA Hand Hygiene Task Force. MMWR; 51(No. RR-16).

- ***Centers for Disease Control and Prevention. Guidelines for infection control in dental healthcare settings*** (2003): Morbid Mortal Wkly Rep MMWR; 52(No. RR17):1- 66.

- ***CDC Guideline for Isolation*** (2004): preventing transmission of Infectious Agent in Health Care Settings Includes the materials from the 2004 Draft. In: Christensen, B.L and Kockrow, E.O (2006): FOUNDATION OF NURSING, Medical /Surgical Asepsis and infection control, Chapter 12, 5th ed, Mosby Elsevire, Pp. 270- 314.

- ***Chandra, S., Bali, R., and Chandra, S.*** (2002): Textbook of pedodontics with 500 multiple choice questions. Infection control and AIDS, 1st ed, Jaypee Brothers Medical Publishers (P) LTD, New Delhi, pp.428- 440.

- ***Christensen, B.L and Kockrow, E.O.*** (2006): Foundation Of Nursing, Medical /Surgical Asepsis and infection control, Chapter 12, 5th ed, Mosby Elsevire, United States of America .Pp. 270- 314.

- ***Cohen, A.S, Jacobsen, E.L, and BeGole, E.A.*** (1997): National survey of endodontists and selected patient samples. Oral Surgery,

Nursing and the challenges toward implementing infection control strategies

Oral Medicine, Oral Pathology, Oral Radiology and Endodontics 83 Pp. 696–702.

- **Cohen, S., and Burns, R.C.** (2002): Pathways of the pulp. Armamentarium and sterilization. Eighth Edition, Mosby, India, Bangladesh P.163, 164.

- **Courtenary, M.A.** (1997): Little knowledge is dangerous thing. Nursing Times July 93 (29): P.67, 78.

- **Craven, R.F, and Hirnle, C.J.** (2007): Fundamentals of Nursing Human Health and Function, 5th ed, Lippincott Williams and Wilkins, Philadelphia .pp 514-545.

- **Danchaivijitr, S., Tantiwatanapaiboon, Y., Chokloikaew, S., Tangtrakool, T., Suttisanon, L., and Chitreechuer, L.** (1995): Universal precautions: knowledge, compliance and attitudes of doctors and nurses in Thailand. J Med Assoc Thai. Jul;78 Suppl 2:S112-7.

- **Daniels, R.** (2004): Nursing Fundamentals Caring and Clinical Decision Making, Infection Control, 1st ed, Thomson Delmar Learning, Australia, Canada .pp 508 -543.

- **Darby, M.L and Walsh, M.M.**(2003): Dental Hygiene Theory and practice, Infection control ,2nd, Saunders, USA, pp.76-108.

- *De almeida, O.P, Scully, C., and Jorges, J.* (1991): Hepatitis B vaccination and infection control in Brazilian dental practice1990. Community Dent Oral Epidemiol; 19(4):225-7.

- *Dement, J.M, Epling, C., Truls, O., Pompeii, L.A., and hunt, D.L.* (2004): Blood and body fluids exposure risks among health care workers. Results from the Duke Health and Safety Surveillance Systems. American Journals of industrial medicine; 46, Pp. 637-648.

- *El Geneidy, M., Okasaha, M., and Oueda, M.* (2000): Infection control in health care settings : "Nurses ethical role " . The fourth international scientific congress. Faculty of Nursing, 332- 353.

- *El -Sayed, H.F, Abaza, S.M, Mehanna S., Winch, P.J.* (1997): The prevalence of hepatitis B and C infections among immigrants to a newly reclaimed area endemic for Schistosoma mansoni in Sinai, Egypt. Acta Tropica, 68:229-237.

- *El-Shenawi, S.H.* (2002): Establishing standards for prevention and control of nosocomial infection in the intensive care unit at Alexandria main University hospital, (unpublished) Doctor Thesis, Alexandria University, Faculty of Nursing.

- *Elewy, E.A.* (1997): Assessment of Nurse's Knowledge Regarding Infection Control precaution at Assiut University Hospital, Thesis Master, Faculty of Nursing. Assiut University. Pp.14-85.

- *El-Shafie, I., Mokabel, F., and Helmy, F.* (1995): The relation ship Between the Knowledge of Nursing staff and their Compliance to

Universal Precaution for Prevention of Hepatitis B Viral Infection. The Journals of Egyptian Public Health Association, LXX56: 523 - 540.

- **Evans, R.** (1989): Acceptance of recommended cross-infection procedures by orthodontists in the United Kingdom. British Journal of Orthodontics 16, Pp. 189–194.

- **Ewen, M.M.** (2002): Community –Based Nursing An introduction, Communicable diseases, 2nd ed, Saunders, Philadelphia, P.451.

- **Fasunloro, A., and Owotade, F.J.** (2004): Occupational Hazards among Clinical Dental Staff. J Contemp Dent Pract (5)2, Pp.134-152.

- **Favero, M.S, Bond, W.W.** (1991): Chemical disinfection of medical and surgical materials. In: Block, S.S., Disinfection, sterilization, and preservation. Philadelphia: Lea and Febiger: 617- 41.

- **Frommer, H.H, and Stabulas-Savage, J.J.** (2005): Infection Control in Dental Practice, Radiology for the dental Professional, Eighth Edition, Elsevier Mosby, United States of America .P.161.

- ***Frotline Health Care Workers National Conferences on Prevention of Sharp Injures and Blood borne Pathogens*** (2000): Washington, DC.

- **Galllab, S.A.** (1994): Development and implementing an Inservice Education Program on Aseptic Techniques and principles of Sterilization for Nurses working in Surgical departments of Assiut

Nursing and the challenges toward implementing infection control strategies

University Hospital, Doctor Thesis, Faculty of Nursing, University of Assiut.

- **Gamal, L.M.** (2005): Establishing standards for prevention and control of nosocomial infection in the Recovery Rooms and Surgical Word at El-Menia University hospital. (Unpublished) Doctor Thesis Faculty of Nursing, University of Assiut.

- **Garner, J.S, and Hospital Infection Control Practices Advisory Committee** (1996): Guideline for isolation precautions in hospitals. Infect Control Hosp Epidemiol; 17:53-80.

- **Gerberding, J.L.** (2003): Clinical practices. Occupational exposure to HIV in health care settings. New England Journals of medicine, 348 (9) .Pp .826-833.

- **Gershon, R.R, Mitchell, C., Sherman, M.F, Vlahov, D., Lears, M.M, Felknor, S., and Lubelczyk, R.A.** (2005): Hepatitis B vaccination in correctional health care workers, Am J Infect Control 33 (9), Pp.510-518.

- **Gilbert, A.D. and Nuttall, N.M.** (1994): Knowledge of the human immunodeficiency virus among final year dental students. Journal of Dentistry; 22, Pp. 229–235.

- **Gluck, G.M and Morganstein, W.M.** (2003): Community Dental Health ,The Impact of Transmissible Diseases On The Practices of Dentistry 5th ed, Mosby, India, pp. 205 -233.

- **Gordon, B.L, Burke F.J, Bagg, J., Marlborough, H.S, and McHugh, S.E.** (2001): Systematic review of adherence to infection control guidelines in dentistry, Journals of Dentistry 29 (8) .pp. 509-516.

- **Green, L. W, and Ottoson, J.M.** (1994): Community Health.7th ed., St Louis: Mosby Co., p.303-318.

- **Gustavo, M., Lara MD, Nemora, T., Sandra, C., and Tudesco, D.S.** (2006): Hepatitis B vaccination in correctional health care workers, American Journals of Infection Control 34 (6).P 399.

- **Hackeny, R., et al.** (1998): Using a biological indicators to detect potential source of cross contamination in the dental operation, J Am Dent Assoc 129:1567.

- **Hassan, A .K.** (2004): Assessment of Health Team Knowledge and Practices about Infection Control in Maternal Child Health Centers in Assiut City. Master Thesis. Faculty of Nursing. Assiut University.

- **Hastreiter, R.J, Roesch, M.H, Danila, R.N, and Falken, M.C.** (1992): Dental health care workers' response to the HIV epidemic. Am J Dent; 5:160-6.

- **Hudson-Davies, S.C, Jones, J.H, and Sarll, D.W.** (1995): Cross-infection control in general dental practice: dentist's behavior compared with their knowledge and opinions, Br Dent J; 178, Pp. 365–369.

- *Health and Welfare Canada. Infection control guidelines for isolation and precaution techniques* (1985): Ottawa: Health and Welfare Canada.

- *Health Canada* (1987): Recommendations for prevention of HIV transmission in health-care settings. CDWR; 13S3:1-10.

- *Health Canada* (1997): Preventing the transmission of blood borne pathogens in health care and public services settings. CCDR; 2353.

- *Henderson, D.K.* (2003): Managing Occupational Risks for Hepatitis C Transmission in the Health Care Setting, Clinical Microbiology Reviews, 16(3), p. 546-568.

- *Huband, S., Trigg, E. and Moores, D.Y.* (2000): Practices in children's Nursing Guideline for Hospital and community. Control of infection, 1st ed, Churchill living stone, Edinburgh, London, Pp.13-27.

- *John, J. H, Thomas, D., Richards, D., and Evans, C.* (2002): Regulating dental nursing in the UK, British Dental Journal; 193(4), pp. 207-209.

- *June, R.P.* (2003): Microbial contamination in dental unit waterlines, Braz. Dent. J;14 (1).

- *Kandeel, A., Talaat, M., El-Shoubary, W., Bodenschatz, C., Khairy I., Oun, S., and Mahoney, F. J.* (2003): Occupational exposure to needle stick injuries and hepatitis B vaccination coverage among health care workers in Egypt, <u>American Journal of Infection Control</u> 31(8), Pp. 469-474.

- **Kane, et al.** (1989): Hepatitis B Infection in United States, Am J Med 87 (suppl 3A) : 11S. In Gluck ,G.M and Morganstein, W.M (2003): Community Dental Health, The Impact of Transmissible Diseases on the Practices of Dentistry, 5th ed, Mosby, India, pp. 205 - 233.

- **Kohn, W., Collins, A., Cleveland, J. , Harte, J., Eklund, K., and Malvitz, D.** (2004): Special Report, Guidelines for infection control in dental health care settings -2003, J Am Dent Assoc;135 (1) pp 33-47.

- **Kretzer, E.K, and Larson E.L.** (1998): Behavioral interventions to improve infection control practices, Am J Infect Control; 26, Pp. 245–253.

- **Lange, P., Savage, N.W, and Walsh, N.J.** (1996): Utilization of personal protective equipment in general dental practice. Australian Dental Journal 41, Pp. 164–168.

- **Larson, E.L, Early, E., Cloonan, P., Sugrue, S., and Parides, M.** (2000): An organizational climate intervention associated with increased Hand washing and decreased nosocomial infections. Behav Med; 26:14-22.

- **Laurenson, I .F, Whyte, A.S, Fox, C., and Babb, J.R.** (1999): Contaminated surgical instruments and variant Creutzfeldt-Jakob disease. Lancet; 354, Pp. 1823-1826.

- *Leahy, J.M, and Kizilay, P.E.* (1998): Foundation of Nursing Practices A Nursing Process Approach, Physiologic and Biologic Safety. The last digit is printed number 9. W.B. Saunders Company, Philadelphia, London .Pp. 400-437.

- *Lipsett, P.A, and Swoboda, S.M.* (2001): Hand washing compliance depends on professional status, Surg Infect 2 ,Pp. 241–245.

- *Lynch, P., Jackson, M.M, and Cummings, M.J, et al.* (1987): Rethinking the role of isolation practices in the prevention of nosocomial infections. Ann Intern Med; 107:243-246.

- *Mahon, R., and Sloan, P.* (2000): Essential of Pathology for Dentistry, Microbes and infection, Churchill living stone, Sydney, Toronto, P.69.

- *Mahoney, F., Stewart, K., Coleman, H. H, and Alter, M.J.* (1997): Progress toward the elimination of hepatitis B virus transmission among health care workers in the United States, Arch Int Med 157 ,pp. 2601–2605.

- *Malik, N.A.* (2002): Text book of Oral and Maxillofacial Surgery, Infection control, 1[st]ed, Jaypee Brothers, New Delh, pp.78-91.

- *Matthews, R.W.* (1989): Attitudes and practices regarding control of cross-infection in general dental practice. Health Trends 21 11–3.

- *Maupomé, G., Borges-Yáñez, S.A, Díez-de-Bonilla, F.J, and Irigoyen-Camacho, M.E.* (2002): Attitudes toward HIV-infected

Nursing and the challenges toward implementing infection control strategies

individuals and infection control practices among a group of dentists in Mexico City-a 1999 update of the 1992 survey, American Journal of infection control; 30 (1) , Pp.8- 14.

- *Mc closkey, J.C and Bulechek, G.M* (2000): Nursing intervention classification (NIC)(3rd). St. Louis :Mosby.

- *Mc Ewen, M.* (2002): Community based Nursing an introduction, Role and Intervention in Community - Based Nursing Practices, 2nd, Saunders, Philadelphia, London .P.20.

- *Mc Neal, G .J.* (2000): AACN Guide to Acute Care Procedure in the home .Infection Control, 20 contributors, Lippincott, Philadelphia .New York, P.26.

- *McCarthy, G.M, and Koval, J.J.* (1996): Changes in dentists' infection control practices, knowledge, and attitudes concerning HIV over a 2-year period. Oral Surg Oral Med Oral Pathol; 81. Pp. 297–302.

- *McCarthy, G.M, and Britton J.E.* (2000): A survey of final-year dental, medical and nursing students: Occupational injuries and infection control, J Can Dent Assoc; 66. pp. 561–565.

- *McCarthy, G.M, and MacDonald, J.K.* (1998): A comparison of infection control practices of different groups of oral specialists and general dental practitioners, Oral Surg Oral Med Oral Pathol Oral Radiol Endod 85, Pp. 47–54.

Nursing and the challenges toward implementing infection control strategies

- *McCarthy, G.M, Koval, J.J, John, M.A, and MacDonald, J.K.* (1999): Infection Control Practices Across Canada: Do Dentists Follow the Recommendations? J Can Dent Assoc. 65, Pp 506 –11.

- *Meengs, M.R, Giles, B.K, Chisholm, C.D, Cordell, W.H, and Nelson, D.R.* (1994): Hand washing frequency in an emergency department. Ann Emerg Med J 23, Pp.1307-12.

- *Meiller, T.F, Kelley, J.I, Baqui, A. A, and DePaola, L.G.* (2000): Disinfection of dental unit waterlines with an oral antiseptic. J Clin Dent; 11:11-15.

- *Michaels, B. Gangar, V. Ayers, T. Meyers, E. and Curiale, M.S.* (2001): The significance of hand drying after hand washing. In: Edwards, J.S, Hewedi M.M, editors. Culinary arts and science III global and national perspectives. Bournemouth (UK): Bournemouth University; p. 294-301.

- *Michalsen, A., Delclos, G.L, Felknor, S.A, Davidson, A.L, Johnson, P.C, and Vesley, D.* (1997): Compliance with universal precautions among physicians, J Occup Environ Med; 39, Pp. 130–137.

- *Miller, C.H, and Palenik, C. J.* (1998): Infection Control and Management of Hazardous Materials for the Dental Team, Chapter Infection control rationales and regulations, Immunization, Protective Barriers, and Instrument processing, 2nd ed, Mosby .St. Lous Baltimore. PP 83-174.

- *Ministry of Health and population, Egypt Infection control Program*, Infection Control Office, and World Health Organization Regional Office for the Eastern Mediterranean. National guidance for infection control " [2]nd part, infection control at different department at heath centers. Pp1-20. http://www.ems.org.eg/esic_home/data/giued_part2/Dentistry.pdf

- *Mitchell, R., and Russell, J.* (1989): The elimination of cross-infection in dental practice- a 5 year follow-up. British Dental Journal 166, Pp. 209–211.

- *Mohammed, A.* (1999): Application of education program for nurses about infection control precaution with Aids and virus hepatitis B, in Assiut university hospital. Pp. 24-29.

- *Molinari, J. A.* (2003): Infection control, its evolution to the current standard precautions, J Am Dent Assoc; 134(5) pp. 569-574.

- *Molinari, J.A.* (1999) *Adapted* (2002): with permission of ADA Business: Dental infection control at the year of 2000. Accomplishment recognized. J Am Den Assoc; 130:1291-1298.

- *Monarca, S., Grottolo, M., Renzi, D., Paganelli, C., Sapelli, P., Zerbini, I., and Nardi, G.* (2000): Evaluation of environmental bacterial contamination and procedures to control cross infection in a sample of Italian dental surgeries. J Occup Environ Med; 57, Pp.721-726.

- *Moore, G., and Griffith, C.J.* (2001): A comparison of traditional and recently developed methods for monitoring surface hygiene within the food industry: a laboratory study. Dairy Food Environ Sanitation; 21:478-88.

- *Morris, E. Hassan, F.S, Al Nafisi, A., and Sugathan, T.N.* (1996): Infection control knowledge and practices in Kuwait: a survey on oral health care workers. Saudi Dent J; 8:19-26.

- *Mousa, A.A, Mahmoud, N.M. and Tag El-Din, A.M.* (1997): Knowledge and attitudes of dental patients towards cross-infection control measures in dental practice, East Mediterr Health J; 3 (2), pp. 263–273.

- *Muawia, A., Qudeimat, B., Razan, Y., Farrah, B ., Arwa, I., and Owais, B.* (2006): Infection control knowledge and practices among dentists and dental nurses at a Jordanian university teaching center, American Journal of Infection Control, 34(4). Pp. 218-222.

- *Murray, C.A, Burke, F.J, and McHugh, S.* (2001): An assessment of the incidence of punctures in latex and non-latex dental examination gloves in routine clinical practice. Br Dent J; 190:377-380.

- *Naidoo, S.* (1997): Dentists and cross-infection: J Dent Assoc S Afr. Mar; 52(3):165-7.

- *Nash, K.D.* (1992): How infection control procedures are affecting dental practice today. J Am Dent Assoc; 123, Pp.67–73.

- *Newman, M.G, Takei, H.H and Carranza, F.A.* (2003): General Principles of periodontal Surgery, clinical periodontology outpatient Surgery, 9th ed, Saunders, Philadelphia, P.726 .

- *NHS Executive* (2000): Decontamination of medical devices. Health Services Circular HSC 2000/032, Department of Health, London.

- *Nies, M.A and Ewen, M.M.* (2001): Community Health Nursing Promoting the Health of Population, Communicable diseases and public health, 3rd ed, W.B Saunders Company. Pp.659-700.

- *NZDA, New Zealand Dental Association* (2002): A joint Code of Practice , Code of Practice Control of Cross Infection in Dental Practice ,pp.1-49.http://www.dentalcouncil.org.nz/Documents/Codes/COP_Infection_Control.pdf.

- *Occupational Safety and Health Administration* (2001): Occupational exposure to blood borne pathogens, needle stick and other sharp injures: Final rule (29 CFR Part 1910, docket no. H370A). Fed Regist ; 66(12):5318-5325.

- *Oeding, M., and Mennito, A.S.* (2005): Infection Control in the Dental Office, Foundation in Continuing Dental Education, Herndon, pp.1-62.

- *Ogden, G.R, Bahrami, M., and Sivarajasingam, V.* (1997): Dental students' knowledge and compliance in cross infection control procedures at a UK dental hospital. Oral Diseases; 3, pp. 25–30.

- **Ogunbodede, E.O.** (1996): Occupational hazards and safety in dental practice. Nigerian J Med; 5, Pp11-15.

- **Phoenix, R.D, Cagna, D.R, DeFreest, C.F.** (2003): Clinical Removable Partial Prosthodontics. Infection control in clinical Prosthodontics, 3rd ed. Quintessence Publishing, Chicago, Berlin. P.136.

- **Pistorius, A., Willershausen, B., and Heffner, N.** (2002): Treatment aspects for patients with infectious diseases in dental practices – results of a survey, Eur J Med Res; 7, Pp. 457–462.

- **Pittet, D.** (2005): Infection control and quality health care in the new millennium, American Journal of Infection Control 33;(5), pp. 258-267.

- **Pittet, D., Mourouga, P., and Perneger, T.M.** (1999): Compliance with hand washing in a teaching hospital, An Internal Med 130, pp. 126-130.

- **Porter, S.R, El-Maaytah, M., Afonso, W., et al.** (1995): Cross infection compliance of UK dental staff and students. Oral Diseases 1, Pp. 198–200.

- **Potter, P.A and Perry, A.G.** (1998): Fundamental of Nursing, Infection Control, Infection control, 4th edition, Mosby, Philadelphia. pp. 533-552.

- ***Potter, P.A, and Perry, A.G.*** (2001): Fundamental of Nursing, Infection Control, Infection control, chapter 33, 5th edition, Mosby, Philadelphia, London .pp .835-882.

- ***Qudeimat, M.A, Farrah ,R. Y, and Owais, A. I.*** (2006): Infection control knowledge and practices among dentists and dental nurses at a Jordanian university teaching center, <u>American Journal of Infection Control</u> ; <u>34 (4)</u>, Pp. 218-222 .

- ***Recommended Infection Control Practices for Dentistry*** (1986): MMWR Morb Mortal Wkly Rep 35:15.

- ***Recommendations for prevention of HIV transmission in health-care settings*** (1987): MMWR Morb Mortal Wkly Rep36:25.

- ***Recommended Infection Control Practices for Dentistry*** (1993): MMWR Morb Mortal Wkly Rep 42: RR-8.

- ***Reis, C., Heisler, M., Amowitz, L.L, Moreland, R.S, Mafeni, J.O, et al.*** (2005): Discriminatory Attitudes and Practices by Health Workers toward Patients with HIV/AIDS in Nigeria. PLoS Med 2(8): 246.

- ***Rogers, B.*** (2003): Occupational and Environmental Health Nursing, Legal Responsibility in Occupational and Environmental Health Nursing Practices, 2nd ed, Saunders An Imprint of Elsevier Science, United States of America, Pp.531-575.

- ***Ryan, K.J, and Ray, C.G.*** (2004): Medical Microbiology an introduction to infectious diseases, Hepatitis viruses, chapter 37, 4th ed, McGRAW-HILL Medical Publishing Division, New York, Pp.541-553.

- **Salamaa, O.E.** (1996): A study of nosocomial infection in general hospital. Journals of the Egyptian Public Health Association ; XXI (1,2): 32- 43.

- **Samarnayake, L.P, Jones, B.M, and Scally, C.** (2002): Essential Microbiology for Dentistry, principles of infection control, 2nd ed, Churchill Livingstone, Edinburgh London, Pp.255-271.

- **Samir, A.A.** (1996): Assessment of Nurses' Knowledge and Practices Regarding Universal Infection Control Precaution of Blood Borne Pathogens. Thesis Master. Alexandria, Egypt. University of Alexandria, Faculty of Nursing.

- **Sarll, D.W, Jones, J.H, and Ashton, M.A.** (1996): Cross-infection control, the role of "in-training" dental nurses, Journal of Dentistry 24(5), Pp.349-353.

- **Scheutz, F., and Langebaek, J.** (1995): Dental care of infectious patients in Denmark, 1986-1993: theoretical considerations and empirical findings. Community Dentistry and Oral Epidemiology; 23, pp. 226–231.

- **Scully, C. Porter, S.R. and Epstein, J.** (1992): Compliance with infection control procedures in a dental hospital clinic, Br Dent J; 173, Pp. 20- 23.

- **Scully, C., and Cawson, A.** (1998): Medical Problems in Dentistry, Medical history and assessment, 4th ed, Wirght, Great Britain, pp.1-12.

- **Sedky, N.A.** (1993): Study of Hepatitis C virus (HCV) Among Dentists In Relation to Infection Control Methods in Alexandria. Thesis Master. Faculty of Dentistry, University of Alexandria.

- **Shahrour, M.S.** (1997): Hepatitis B among dental personnel. Evaluation of their knowledge, attitudes and behaviors. Eastern Mediterranean Health Journals 3 (3):549-555.

- **Shulman, E.R and Brehm, W.T.** (2001): Dental clinical attire and infection-control procedures, J Am Dent Assoc; 132(4) pp. 508-516.

- **Silverman, S., Eversole, L.R, and Truelove, E.L.** (2001): Essential of oral medicine. Infection control, 1st ed, BC Decker Inc, London, pp180-185.

- **Smeltzer, S.C and Bare, B. G.** (2004): Text book of Medical Surgical Nursing, 10th ed, Management of patient with infectious diseases, chapter 70, Lippincott Williamms and Wilkins, Philadelphia, pp. 2114-2125 .

- **Smitch, C.M, and Maurer, F.A.** (1995): Community Health Nursing Theory and Practices. Contemporary Problems in Community Health Nursing, W.B. Saunders Company, Philadelphia, London. P.474.

- *Snyder, G.A.* (1993): Pennsylvania dental hygienists knowledge, attitudes and infection control practices in relation to AIDS and AIDS patients. Journal of Dental Hygiene; 67, Pp. 188-196.

- *Sproat, L.J, and Inglis, T.J.* (1994): A multi center survey of hand hygiene practice in intensive care units. J Hosp Infect; 26, Pp.137-48.

- *Stein, A. D, Makarawo, T. P, and Ahmad, M. F.* (2003): A survey of doctors' and nurses' knowledge, attitudes and compliance with infection control guidelines in Birmingham teaching hospitals, Journal of Hospital Infection 54 (1), Pp. 68-73.

- *Talaat, M., Kandeel, A., Rasslan, O., Hajjeh, R., Hallaj, Z., El-Sayed, N., and Mahoney, F.J.* (2003): Evolution of infection control in Egypt: Achievements and challenges, American Journal of Infection Control,34(4), Pp 193-200.

- *Tarantola, A., Abiteboul, D., and Rachline, A.* (2006): Infection risks following accidental exposure to blood or body fluids in healthcare workers: A review of pathogens transmitted in published cases. American Journal of Infection Control; 34(6) pp.367-375.

- *Thompson, B.L, Dwyer, D.M, Ussery , X.T, Denman, S., Vacek , P., and Schwartz, B.* (1997): Hand washing and glove use in a long term care facility, Infect Control Hosp Epidemiol; 18, Pp. 97-103.

- *Toukan, A.* (1997): Control of hepatitis B in the Middle East. In : Rizzetto M, ed. proceeding of IX triennial international symposium of

Viral Hepatitis and liver disease. turin, Edizioni Minerva Medica :678-9.

- **Trapé-Cardoso, M., and Schenck, P.** (2004): Reducing percutaneous injuries at an academic health center: A 5-year review, Am J Infect Control 32(5), Pp. 301-305.

- **Treasure, E.T, and Treasure, P.** (1997): Investigation of the disposal of hazardous wastes from New Zealand dental practices. Community Dentistry and Oral Epidemiology Journals; 25, Pp. 328–331.

- **UNAIDS US Census Bureau, Ministry of Health and Population National AIDS Program:** (2005). http://www. synergyaids. com/Profiles _Web/Profiles_ PDFs / EgyptProfileFINAL2005.pdf

- **Update: Universal precaution for prevention transmission of HIV, HBV, and other blood borne pathogens in health care settings** (1988): MMWR Morb Mortal Wkly Rep37:24.

- **US Department of health and human services** (2000): Healthy people 2010: Conference edition . Washington. DC.

- **US Department of Labor, Occupational Safety and Health Administration** (2001): 29 CFR Part 1910.1030. Occupational exposure to blood borne pathogens; needle stick and other sharps injuries; final rule. Federal Register; (66):5317- 3525.

- *USPHS, DHHS, and CDC* (2003): Healthcare Infection Control Practices Advisory Committee, draft guideline for environmental infection control in health care facilities, Publications 97-135.

- *Vignarajah, S., Eastmond ,V.H , Ashraph, A., and Rashad, M.* (1998): An assessment of Cross- infection control procedures among English - Speaking Caribbean general dental practitioners. A regional preliminary study. International dental Journals 48(1), Pp. 67-76.

- *Walsh, L.J, Lange, P., and Savage, N.W.* (1995): Factors influencing the wearing of protective gloves in general dental practice. Quintessence International; 26, Pp. 203–209.

- *Weightman, N.C, and Lines, L.D.* (2004): Problems with the decontamination of dental handpieces and other intra-oral dental equipment in hospitals, Journals of Hospital Infection, 56(1), Pp.1-5.

- *While, L. and Duncan, G.* (2002): Medical Surgical Nursing .An International approach, 2nd ed, Califton Park, NY: Delmar Learning.

- *WHO* (2003): Practical Guideline For Infection Control In Health Care Facilities, p. 9.

- *WHO.* Grant NO.EN/90/06545. In *Sedky, N.A.* (1993): Study of Hepatitis C virus (HCV) Among Dentists In Relation to Infection Control Methods in Alexandria. Thesis Master. Faculty of Dentistry, University of Alexandria.

- *Wilson, T.G and kornman, K.S.* (2003): Infection control and Personnel Safety, fundamental of Periodontics, 2nd ed, Quintessence Publishing Co, Chicago, pp.238-254.

- *Wiwanitkit, V.* (2006): Blood borne viral pathogens and the feasibility of passing thorough the gloves: An appraisal and implication on infection control. <u>American Journal of Infection Control</u>, 34 (6), P .400.

- *Wong, C.* (2003): Prevention of spread of infection in dental practice, Oral Implants, An official quarterly publication of Hong Kong society of implantlogy with technical support by Asian implantlogy Center; 8 (2).

- *Wood, P.J.* (1995): Infection control practices of Rhode Island Dental Hygienists and Certified Dental Assistants. Journal of Dental Hygiene (69), pp. 212–222.

- *World Health Organization Regional Office for the Eastern Mediterranean* (1995): Intercountry workshop on the prevention and control of viral hepatitis. Alexandria. In *Qirbil, N., and Hall, A.J.* (2001): Epidemiology of hepatitis B virus infection in the Middle East, Eastern Mediterranean   Health Journals 7(6), p .1035.

- *World Health reports* (1998): Repot of the director-general, Geneva: World Health Organization.

- *World Health Organization* (2001): AIDS in the Eastern Mediterranean Region (2000): Progress report, EMRO. Cairo, Eastern Mediterranean Regional Office, (Em/RC 47/INF.DOC.2).

- *World Health Organization Report* (2002): Prevention of hospital-acquired infections. A practical guide. 2nd edition. WHO/CDS/CSR/ EPH/2002.12

- *Wray, D., Stenhouise, D., Lee, D., and Clark, A. J.* (2003): Text book of general and oral surgery. Cross -infection, 1st ed, Churchill living stone, London. PP. 46-53.

- *Younai, F.S, Murphy, D.C, and Kotelchuck, D.* (2001): Occupational exposures to blood in a dental teaching environment: results of a ten-year surveillance study. J Dent Educ; (65):436-438.

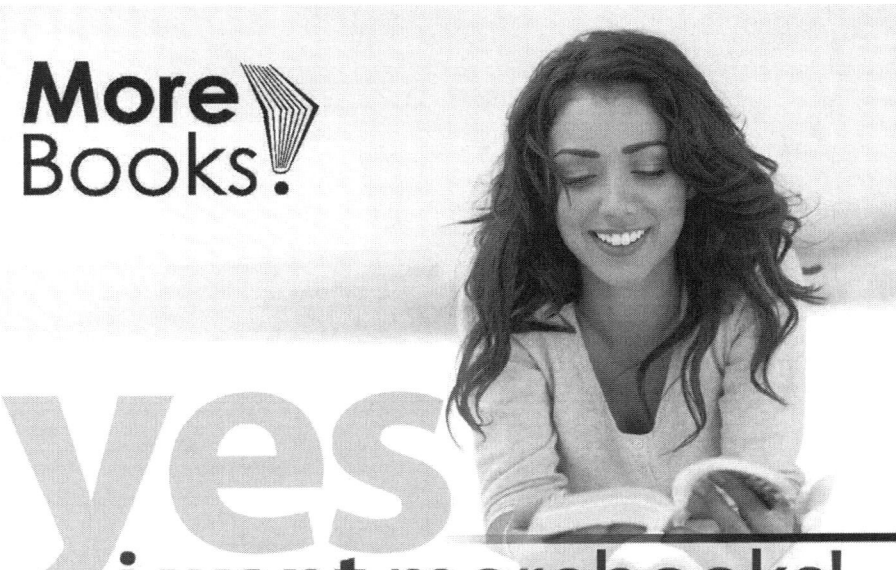
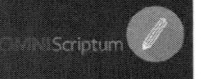

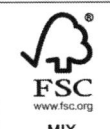

Druck:
Canon Deutschland Business Services GmbH
im Auftrag der KNV-Gruppe
Ferdinand-Jühlke-Str. 7
99095 Erfurt